ALSO BY MAGGIE & NIGEL PERCY

The Nature Of Intuition: Understand & Harness Your Intuitive Ability

The Busy Person's Guide To Energy Clearing

The Busy Person's Guide To Ghosts, Curses & Aliens

The Busy Person's Guide To Space Clearing

The Busy Person's Guide: The Complete Series

Dowsing For Health: Awaken Your Hidden Talent

101 Amazing Things You Can Do With Dowsing

Dowsing Ethics: Replacing Intentions With Integrity

Dowsing: Practical Enlightenment

The Dowsing State: Secret Key To Accurate Dowsing

Ask The Right Question: The Essential Sourcebook Of Good Dowsing
Questions

The Dowsing Encyclopedia

The Essence Of Dowsing by Nigel Percy

The Credibility Of Dowsing, edited by Nigel Percy

Healing Made Simple: Change Your Mind & Improve Your Health

Caring For Your Animal Companion

THE BUSY PERSON'S GUIDE TO NATURAL HEALTH

BUSY PERSON'S GUIDES, BOOK 5

MAGGIE PERCY

NIGEL PERCY

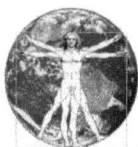

In questions of science, the authority of a thousand is not worth the humble reasoning of a single individual.

- Galileo Galilei

CONTENTS

Preface   ix
Acknowledgments   xv
Introduction   xvii
How To Use This Guide   xxi
Warning   xxiii

1. What Is Natural Health?   1
2. Is Medical Science Always Right?   13
3. Health Goals & Paradigms   20
4. Physical Health Factors   25
5. Mental, Emotional & Energetic Health Factors   52
6. Technology's Dangers   65
7. Taking Action   89
8. It's Your Choice   121
9. Using Dowsing & Intuition   131
10. Summary   134
11. Resources   136

Please Leave A Review   147
Other Busy Person's Guides   149
About Maggie & Nigel Percy   151

PREFACE

This could be one of the most important books you ever read, but it will challenge you. We are going to ask you to step back and look at health in a new way, and it may not be easy for you to do that, because it will take a conscious effort, and you will need to think critically. Yet that is how you open yourself to solutions to your health problems and learn how to create the health you desire.

You can't create success by doing things the same way you've always done them. This guide will give you a new framework for creating the health you want, and if you are able to keep an open mind, it will do so rather quickly.

It took me nearly thirty years of seeking, learning and thinking to form this approach, and I believe it will help kick start your health journey and set you on a good path. But that doesn't mean this guide has all the answers. Indeed, I am still seeking a better understanding of health, because in thirty years what I have learned best is that there is much yet to be discovered about how good health is created.

Like everyone, I have always been amazed at the great strides in science and technology during my lifetime. I have two degrees in Biology, and I was taught to revere the scientific method and to accept what Science says is 'truth.' (Science with a capital 'S' meaning the scientific establishment that preaches certain facts as infallible).

I graduated from college in 1974, and yet, since that time, there have been many scientific discoveries that have forced the scientific establishment to reverse itself on the very subjects I was taught were rock solid truths. When I took my courses in genetics, the human genome had not been mapped, nor did epigenetics exist as a field of study. We now know that genetic expression is far more flexible than was preached in the 20th century, but sadly, medicine doesn't seem to have caught up with this fact, and still wants you to think your genes are your destiny.

Nature vs. Nurture (do genes or the environment matter more) was a very hot topic in Biology when I was in college, and now we know that it isn't either/or. Because so little was known, each side was speculating; each side was able to make a case for their point of view. In the end, the bigger picture showed that the whole controversy was pointless. Both sides were right. The environment and your genes work together in very complex ways to help you live a more healthy life.

There have been many other reversals of scientific dogma in my lifetime, and most of them were because conclusions were drawn with incomplete evidence. To illustrate, think about how, when I was a child, acupuncture was believed to be a bunch of hooey by the scientific establishment, because it was virtually unknown in the US. Now, many allopathic doctors are on board with it as a therapy. Ayurveda for thousands of years said the brain has a lymphatic system, but traditional medicine denied it until 2015 when it was 'proven' to exist. Now traditional medicine accepts it, but you won't hear them saying they made a mistake all those years they denied it existed.

One of the most important, foundational facts, which will be repeated throughout the guide is this: we actually are amazingly ignorant of human biology and how to create good health, no matter what the scientific establishment would have you believe. That there is a huge amount of undiscovered knowledge explains the many reversals of dogma, not just during my life, but throughout history.

As in the fable of the blind men and the elephant, scientists are often carried away by the excitement of discovery and draw sweeping conclusions without enough evidence to support them. Later, as more knowledge is gathered, new theories are formed and old ones are discarded, because that is the nature of pure science. A true scientist wants to know and keeps seeking knowledge, formulating theories and testing them.

The problem is that the scientific establishment is wedded to particular theories, disregarding that they are merely theories, and clings to them way past the time when new facts have come to light showing them to be faulty. Eventually, those theories fall apart and are replaced, but when those attitudes and practices have to do with medicine and public health, people can be harmed in the meantime.

Years ago, we were told free radicals are awful, and we should get rid of them, so we invested in supplements to fight free radicals, then not so many years later, we were told you need a certain amount of free radicals, and it's dangerous to wipe them all out. For many years, we were told 'germs' are bad for you, and we should kill them with antibacterial soaps, cleaners and drugs. Now the establishment is admitting there are 'good' bacteria, but they haven't stopped the wholesale assault on microorganisms, and it is leading to bad consequences. Healthy fats and cholesterol were major health topics for years. Margarine was pushed on people as a 'healthy' replacement for butter; now butter is back in, and at least some doctors admit cholesterol is vital for manufacturing hormones. Not only do the reversals seem almost laughable; think of the cost of false dogmas to the public in terms of money and health.

Maybe it would be wiser to admit we don't know everything, and that Science, which focuses on a reductionistic approach (breaking things down into smaller and smaller parts as a way of gaining knowledge), has yet to plumb the complex connections between the various parts of your body, the environment and your thoughts, emotions and beliefs. There is so much to learn, and that knowledge is bound to overturn many long-held scientific beliefs.

Knowing that we just don't know everything is key to understanding and making good health choices, because admitting ignorance gives you a hungry mind that is open to new information and ideas. That is the first step in our approach to natural health.

So what do you do when you are basically unaware of all you need to know about how your body works or what it needs to be healthy? Ask what Nature has shown to be true and use that as a guide in making choices, because Mother Nature doesn't make mistakes. Ask what has been proven by the test of evolutionary time and let it be your guide.

The approach in this guide suggests that you alter your thinking to avoid just doing whatever the medical establishment says, because current medical practice has wandered far from what is natural, instead embracing technology, chemicals and surgery as the main ways to cure ill health, and all of its rigid tenets are based on a fraction of the knowledge we need to understand in order to create good health. We do not consider this a formula for success.

To get perspective, ask yourself: how often are accepted medical practices really curing anything? Obesity, cancer, diabetes, autism and Alzheimer's are on the rise, which would seem to argue that we are going in the wrong direction if what we seek is good health. Shouldn't our society be healthier rather than sicker if modern medical science is correct in its approach? What's to blame? We think it is a faulty outlook and arrogance in some cases combined with greed, but regardless of the answer, you don't need to be stuck in a failed health paradigm.

In this guide, we show you an approach that will help you avoid unfortunate and even deadly choices for your health and well-being. You don't have to be a scientist or doctor to easily see the fallacy in bad arguments. You don't have to do tons of research to know when an agenda is being pushed that may harm you and your loved ones and is based on profit as a motive. You don't have to have medical training or a degree in Biology to make smart, empowered choices. You just need to have a few tools, and this guide provides them.

Maggie Percy

April 2019

Addendum, December 2025:

In the past six years, much has happened. I unpublished this book during the pandemic to avoid Amazon pulling it or our other titles on the basis of content that was being censored. I am republishing it now, because even though the past six years has brought some changes to my personal perspective on natural health, I believe the content is useful as a basis for taking responsibility for your own health. Please consult the resources for suggestions that will allow you to take this further.

ACKNOWLEDGMENTS

I want to thank my husband and co-author Nigel for tirelessly editing what I wrote in this guide, so that readers could have a pleasant and clear reading experience. Furthermore, his suggestions strengthened the message tremendously by helping me make it more coherent, consistent and logical.

I am so grateful for my wonderful advance readers, who pointed out remaining errors so that I could fix them before launch day. Without their help, the final product would have not been as smooth and polished. A special thanks to Bernice and Jody for pointing out multiple errors that slipped by our editing. We are blessed to have such a great team!

INTRODUCTION

It's important to start from a shared understanding of terms, so this guide starts by defining what we mean by natural health. Then, building on that foundation, we lay the groundwork for how you can create a successful program of natural health in your life, one that will work for you, your family and your pets.

You may be expecting a list of dos and don'ts, but that's not what this guide is. Modern life is changing so fast that any list will quickly become obsolete.

Instead, the goal of this guide is to give you a framework for making healthy choices in any situation. It doesn't guarantee you won't make mistakes, but it does assure your results will be better than if you just follow the crowd. Modern health care has been harnessed by corporations to generate profit, and that motive does not always line up with your health goals, so it behooves you to make your own choices.

We live in exciting times, where old models of health are being questioned, new theories and facts are emerging to support ancient healing methods, and the body is being regarded as not just a machine, but a complex organism comprised of many parts that supports interactions within itself and with the environment in amazing ways to create balance and harmony.

We are awakening to the realization that we simply don't understand very much about human health and biology. We are learning exciting facts like food and light are information for the body, not just fuel, and that thoughts have a huge impact on physical health.

The new information, which is coming in at a frenetic pace, requires a complete rethinking of the whole subject of human biology and how to create good health. We are modifying a 17th century model based on classical physics into a sleek, 21st century model based on quantum physics. The outcome is stunning, in that it shows that many ancient techniques and teachings about health are in alignment with a quantum-based model. Who knew? Maybe you did in your heart, and now there are finally studies to back up your intuition.

This guide draws on cutting edge science and combines it with ancient wisdom in a straightforward fashion to allow you to be open to the changing health paradigm and to be capable of integrating new discoveries into a coherent health program. Bear in mind two things: there is no single program or silver bullet for health, because each person is unique; and, we only know a small percent of all there is to learn about health, so it behooves us to be open to new ideas and to question everything. In this guide, we acknowledge that and show you how to make better health choices as a result.

The Busy Person's Guides do not go in depth on background research, but rather, give you actionable suggestions for quickly becoming competent to create the outcomes you desire. The Resources will list some material if you want to dive deeper into this important subject.

All of the suggestions in this book are based on extensive research by the authors. If you wish, you can google any of the concepts in this book, and if you look carefully, you will find plenty to support what is suggested, although you will also discover controversy and skepticism. By using your powers of intuition and critical thinking, you can navigate through the masses of information, extracting what is most in alignment with your viewpoint and goals.

In this guide, I draw on my education (two degrees in Biology), my work experience (as a scientific researcher at NASA and as an energy worker and dowser) and what I have learned on my own healing journey since 1990 to give you a jump start on creating the health you want.

Warning: This guide will present ideas that can be regarded as frightening or overwhelming. That is not our intention. Don't try to absorb all the material too quickly. Don't try to change too much, too fast. Take your time.

Think of natural health as growing a garden. Plant seeds, flow with the seasons and do whatever is appropriate for creating a bountiful harvest, and be aware that although there are guidelines for success, each garden is unique, each climate is unique and each plant species is unique, just as each gardener is unique.

You are embarking on a journey of self-discovery and consciousness that is therefore unique to you. Be patient and enjoy the process. Use your heart and your intuition as much as you use your head to make the best decisions for you.

Final note from the authors: This guide is larger than the other three in our *Busy Person's Guides* series, because it is a far more complex topic, even when handled in as concise a way as possible. In the other guides, we present action items for dealing with phenomena you are at least already prepared to understand and believe. Natural health requires a reboot of your perspective, so we have included facts and quotations that we found helpful in this regard. Before you can benefit from what we suggest, you need to fine tune your viewpoint. If you are already on board with this outlook, it will be good reinforcement; if you are new to natural health, it will help you focus on new ways to regard health.

The other *Busy Person's Guides* run from 20-25K words each. This one will require a little more time to complete and digest.

HOW TO USE THIS GUIDE

The Busy Person's Guides are designed to help you become competent quickly in a given subject, without the fluff and filler you'd get in a full-length book. The exercises are designed to get you thinking and help you learn faster.

The Busy Person's Guide To Natural Health is not a comprehensive book on the topic of natural health, nor is it a complete course in the subject. Instead, it is meant to quickly orient you with the basics and give you the foundation for making wise health choices using a natural perspective.

Using your own natural ability to think critically is vital in creating good health, because we simply don't know all there is to know about human biology, and it is a mistake to become brainwashed by whatever beliefs the medical establishment is promoting at any given time, because as we have pointed out, over time they reverse themselves frequently. To create the health you want, you need to be able to ask good questions, think logically and have some way of evaluating your options. Our goal is to help you be able to do this.

In order to get the most of this guide, you need to read it in its entirety. The point of the guide is to help you have a good basic grounding in as many important natural health subjects as possible, and to teach you how to view things from a natural perspective, and to do that, one chapter builds on another. There will be a small amount of repetition to help you remember key points.

It is possible to get through the guide in one intensive weekend, but you will probably absorb the material better if you spread it out over a month. You need to spend less than ten or fifteen minutes a day to complete the guide in that time.

Do all the exercises and think about what you have read. If at the end of the book, you are enthusiastic about pursuing health in a natural way, start using the Resources section to begin deeper research.

Remember, we know so little of what there is to know about human biology, and more is being discovered every day, upsetting the current health paradigm and proving the wisdom of ancient health systems. Be open to new ideas as well as new facts. You will never learn it all, but if you keep seeking, you will learn enough to make a difference in your health and that of your loved ones.

This guide is longer than each of the three other guides in the series because of the breadth of material it has to cover. Since your time is valuable, we haven't filled the book with references and anecdotes, but there are a few to help punctuate important points.

Each topic in this guide is worthy of a full book of its own, so please do not assume that what you have learned here is everything. But when you put it all together, the content of this guide forms a compelling argument for a more holistic and natural view of health.

WARNING

This guide is intended to give you information to stimulate thought and further research on your part. We trust you to make good choices for your health. Make sure that you take the time to get a second and third opinion and to research important topics fully before making important health choices. This guide is only a starting point for thinking in new ways. It does not purport to be comprehensive, nor is it a complete course.

This guide is not intended to replace the advice of your chosen health care professional. We all need outside help at times. We advise you to select doctors who support your participation in the healing process, who treat you with respect and listen to what you say. It doesn't matter whether you go the holistic or conventional route as long as you stick to those principles. You are the one who has the most to lose or gain concerning your health; you have a right to participate fully in creating the health you want.

If you find this topic intriguing, the Resources section gives you a jumping off point for further research, but it doesn't pretend to be complete. There are so many new resources appearing almost daily that we urge you to pay attention and look for new information and data at all times. You will have to use your judgment about whom to follow.

No one has the complete picture. No one will in our lifetime. That's really the fun of being a scientist: discovering new things and new concepts. We urge you to adopt a true scientific position and question everything and look forward to new bits of useful information in seeing the big picture of how health is created. By going back to the basics of natural health, you won't be led wrong, and you will enhance your results for your health goals.

1

WHAT IS NATURAL HEALTH?

What is natural health? Definitions vary slightly, but all refer to the assumption that the body's natural state is balance, harmony and good health, and that if the body becomes unbalanced, natural remedies and therapies exist that can gently and safely help the body to restore harmony and good health.

This is very different from the basis of modern medicine, which does not assign any particular intelligence or healing ability to the human body. Instead, the body is regarded as a machine. The basis of this concept came from 17th Century physics and philosophy.

The 20th Century gave birth to quantum physics, which challenges the old ways of thinking, but even in the 21st Century, the tenets of quantum physics are being used mainly in holistic and alternative healing systems, and those are based on ancient wisdom, which strangely, aligns beautifully with quantum physics.

Natural health is of course based on Nature. Nature is very much a 'big picture' subject. It is impossible to explore Nature without becoming aware of how much we don't know about how it works. The complexity and beauty of Nature inspires awe and respect.

Natural health is based on that 'big picture' outlook and a respect for Nature as well as the understanding that we know so very little about how it works. Nature is our wise teacher, not something to be scoffed at for being 'primitive' and 'unscientific.'

Natural health has gained many adherents, to the point that in the US, the establishment has passed laws forcing people to belong to the allopathic health care system, because it is failing dramatically and people are fleeing it for holistic, natural methods. This health revolution began decades ago and will continue for the foreseeable future, and you will need to choose which perspective to follow. Your health and well-being may depend on it.

In this guide we will give you tools for making choices that align with natural health to whatever degree you choose to follow it.

~

Your Body Can Heal Itself

Natural health is based on the belief that the body is designed to function well and be healthy, and that when it gets out of balance and experiences dis-ease, it can usually be restored to balance and proper function using natural methods, meaning things found in nature. Of course, it is understood that the more out of balance the system becomes, the more work it takes to restore balance, and sometimes major trauma requires extreme intervention to avert death.

Modern medicine is new, historically speaking. It was only in the 20th Century in the US that the current allopathic establishment set about eliminating other medical methods and perspectives via legislation and smear campaigns. Methods like homeopathy (which the Queen of England uses), chiropractic and osteopathy were painted as quack medicine, establishing allopathy as the primary medical paradigm. Yet in the US, all of these 'alternative' methods are experiencing a resurgence as people turn away from allopathic medicine in search of cures for their ailments.

We advocate natural health as the safest, most effective way to heal your body and restore balance and harmony. If you accept that the body has an amazing capacity to heal itself given the right ingredients and circumstances, then you are ready to use natural health to your advantage.

Modern science is finally supporting these assumptions with actual evidence. It has taken a long time, because throughout the 20th Century and into the current century, reductionism and the mechanical view of the human body dominated research. In other words, scientists took things apart to understand how they worked instead of looking at systems as a whole. For example, they wanted to find the 'active ingredient' in a herb that had long been successfully used for healing, as if the whole herb wasn't of interest, so they paid big money to tear the plant apart and find one or two compounds that could be patented and sold as 'cures,' because whole plants cannot be patented. But the whole plant *was* the cure, and limiting a drug to a big dose of one or two synthetic compounds did not improve on Mother Nature. It created side effects for the sake of profit.

Another example is in the field of genetics. Scientists looked at DNA as the final word in heritability when I was in college, but then the human genome project proved genes weren't enough to explain the diversity and volume of activities going on biologically, and the field of epigenetics was born, demonstrating that genes respond to many environmental factors that change their expression, and those changes can even be passed on to future generations. Yet even now, doctors are 'selling' genetics tests and convincing people to act in fear as if all genes are expressed or expressed the same way. In doing so, they are driven by profit, not science, because epigenetics proves that there are many factors that turn genes on and off. That is what scientists should be looking at, and one day, hopefully, they will.

Reductionism in science is reversing, with more scientists looking at 'the big picture' of how things work rather than breaking things down into component parts. It turns out that the human body is an amazing, complex organism, and we understand so little of what is going on in it and how it relates to health. Being aware of that ignorance allows us to be open to seeing things in new ways, ways that can lead to better health outcomes.

~

Your Body Is A Small Universe

The new biology is focused on systems and how they interact, on how environment stimulates reactions in living organisms, on how the whole is greater than the sum of its parts. This attitude aligns with the perspectives that gave birth thousands of years ago to ancient healing systems like Ayurveda and Traditional Chinese Medicine.

Energy of all kinds is becoming an acknowledged part of health. Meridians, acupuncture and chakras are no longer woo-woo subjects, but are useful for explaining observed quantum phenomena. Emotional trauma and stress are proven factors in the dis-ease process.

The science of epigenetics proves your genes aren't your destiny, that your environment determines a lot about health, and that changes in genes due to environmental factors can be passed on to future generations. It isn't just mutation that changes genes; in fact, that is a minimal aspect of genetic change. Your thoughts, trauma, what you eat, drink and breathe all affect genetic expression.

The body has been shown to be a universe, an ecological system that includes not only trillions of human cells that make up organs and systems, but millions of nonhuman microorganisms that make up the microbiome of the human skin and digestive tract. Without these tiny creatures' help, humans cannot survive, or at least, they don't thrive.

We are learning that we are closely connected with everything else. For example, microRNAs are present in the food we eat. (MicroRNAs are a subset of RNA. RNA is a messenger from DNA that regulates the genome and controls the synthesis of proteins which are essential for virtually everything happening in our body, from the structure of our bodies to holding our genetic code. The term for this activity is gene expression.) When we consume the food, the MicroRNAs enter our blood and alter our gene expression. Sayer Ji, a natural health expert, says,

> Basically, we're finding that over the course of evolution we have literally outsourced gene regulation to the plants in our environment, and also there's other passengers on this journey with us. Bacteria produce microRNAs, for example. And they help to orchestrate the complexity of our being... there is interspecies communication occurring through the mechanism of MicroRNAs, such that the biosphere is actually all one, on some basic molecular level.

Furthermore, microbiologist Kiran Krishnan says,

> We've got 150 times more bacterial and viral DNA in our body than human DNA. It's looking like 99% of metabolic function, things that we do on a daily basis that make us human, are coded for by bacterial and viral DNA. We can barely do anything for ourselves. We need the microbial DNA to conduct necessary functions to live, to digest food, to breathe. Even how our emotions and view of the world are concentrated and how they're characterized are dependent on the types of microbes and microbial DNA we have in our system... We're really a walking, talking ecology. We're like a walking, talking rainforest. There's a massive amount of structure to the ecology. Different parts of the body, different ecologies within the

body have to communicate with one another. We require all of their help in order to be human.

Empowerment is part of the natural health movement. If it is true that the body has the capacity to heal and that Nature provides tools for restoring good health, then you can make choices that encourage health, that restore balance and harmony and that help you achieve your health goals by aligning with Nature's time-tested design.

～

The Test Of Time

Natural health is based on the observed fact that eons of time have shaped organisms to survive and thrive in their natural environments. Evolutionary biology studies the factors that have shaped all living things. Predictable factors in a natural environment, like day length, become key triggers for important biological functions. Unpredictable factors in an environment, like a volcano exploding or a sudden climatic shift, shape adaptations and select for certain responses that get passed on epigenetically as well as via mutations.

Humans are not the only species that experience this process. Every species on earth is subject to it. The upshot is that over great periods of time, like millions of years, a species falls into a give-and-take interaction with the important factors in the environment that affect overall health and reproductive success. In being shaped by these factors, a species develops a dynamic collaboration with the environment that is optimal for health and well-being, even to the point of becoming dependent on other species for survival. To learn about health, it is useful to understand the environmental factors that affect health and that have become encoded in the process over millennia.

Natural health is based on eons of time that have shaped how human health is created. When you test anything for whether it is natural, you will ask who made it (man or Nature), how long has that thing or process been around, and has it passed the test of eons of time in terms of being safe and effective? If it is manmade or has only been around for a hundred years, it is not natural or proven safe. That does not mean it is automatically bad or dangerous; it means that you would be wise to invest some time in questions and critical thinking before blindly adopting new, manmade techniques or 'cures.' In this book, we are going to propose that time is a far better judge of what works than a couple of scientific studies. As Michael Crichton says in his novel, *Prey:*

> If we were to grasp the true nature of nature—if we could comprehend the real meaning of evolution—then we would envision a world in which every living plant, insect, and animal species is changing at every instant, in response to every other living plant, insect and animal. Whole populations of organisms are rising and falling, shifting and changing. This restless and perpetual change, as inexorable and unstoppable as the waves and tides, implies a world in which all human actions necessarily have uncertain effects. The total system we call the biosphere is so complicated that we cannot know in advance the consequences of anything that we do.

> That is why even our most enlightened past efforts have had undesirable outcomes—either because we did not understand enough, or because the ever-changing world responded to our actions in unexpected ways. From this standpoint, the history of environmental protection is as discouraging as the history of environmental pollution...

> The fact that the biosphere responds unpredictably to our actions is not an argument for inaction. It is, however, a powerful argument for caution, and for adopting a tentative attitude toward all we believe, and all we do. Unfortunately, our species has demonstrated a

striking lack of caution in the past. It is hard to imagine that we will behave differently in the future.

We think we know what we are doing. We have always thought so. We never seem to acknowledge that we have been wrong in the past, and so might be wrong in the future. Instead, each generation writes off earlier errors as the result of bad thinking by less able minds— and then confidently embarks on fresh errors of its own.

What the human body has evolved to use over time are the tried and true ways to go. You can add 'modern' manmade methods after reviewing them carefully, if you conclude they are safe. Change is inevitable biologically. But a cautious plan is not to make radical, unnatural changes to a system that has become balanced over many thousands, even millions, of years.

~

Nature Cures

What does nature provide that contributes to good health? Simple things like sunlight, pure water, fresh air, cooperative microorganisms and nutritious food. Living in a crowded, hermetically sealed environment is a new development for humans that deprives the body of sunlight and fresh air, two vital factors for good health. Fear of 'germs' has created aversion to dirt, which contains microorganisms that help us adapt and build strong immune systems. Processed and genetically altered food has replaced proper food, leading to not only digestive problems, but other physical and even mental issues. A sedentary lifestyle robs humans of the chance to move the body, which is also a part of good health.

Nature is your ally. Sunlight and food are your friends. In fact, natural dirt is your friend. If you have food allergies, autoimmune disease or frequently are ill, you have gotten out of the balance your body needs, and you may need to temporarily eliminate certain things to allow your body to heal, but your best overall goal is to restore the natural balance to your body so it can function as it was intended to in and by Nature.

There are circumstances where extreme intervention is needed to restore health, or at least to prevent death, but that fact does not refute the power of natural cures. In a later chapter, we will point out steps that allow you to take advantage of the free natural processes that support good health.

∾

Natural Health For Animals

Your pets, animal companions and livestock have been selectively bred for traits that are not common in Nature, and in fact, most domesticated animals cannot survive well, or at all, on their own. This is because we humans have chosen to create life forms for our own purposes that don't have the benefit of millions of years of evolutionary history and testing. These animals are thus reliant on us for good health.

When humans first experimented with selective breeding, wild animals were modified to make them better food sources or more valuable servants. Because optimal longevity is not a concern in animals raised for food, and because profit was important, natural feeding, housing and care were not deemed worthy of investment. Even in animals not raised for food, such as horses, donkeys and other beasts of burden, there was little motivation to invest in creating optimal longevity, as elderly animals cost money to feed and couldn't pull their own weight, and most people simply did not have the money to support retired animals.

The predictable outcome of this pattern was less humane living conditions for livestock and farm animals. Yet that trend is now reversing. Feedlots for cattle, giant milking barns with cows attached to machines and chickens tightly crowded into metal buildings are being rejected as unacceptable environments by enlightened consumers. Whether they object to the karma of mistreating animals who end up being dinner or they are aware that stress, trauma and poor nutrition create less healthy food, people are moving away from factory farming.

It isn't only livestock who benefit from a more natural lifestyle; pets live longer, healthier and happier lives if given what Nature intended for them.

Regardless of how much domesticated species have changed from their wild cousins, certain truths apply. If you want your animal companion or farm animals to be healthy, provide them with as close to a natural life as you can. That means feed them a natural diet, not processed foods. Give them exercise and safe access to the outdoors. And avoid overuse of unnatural things like drugs, vaccines and chemicals.

Some examples of unnatural choices that contribute to ill health include:

- Vegetarian diets for cats and dogs (who are carnivores)
- Feeding cheap, highly processed foods devoid of enzymes, minerals and microorganisms
- Keeping horses penned up in barn stalls and feeding them too much grain (instead of letting them roam and graze all day in the sunshine)
- Chemically worming, vaccinating frequently and using drugs (these further stress the body and have toxicity and other side effects that impact health)

Unnatural living creates stress which leads to imbalance and disease. A good example is found in horses. Anyone who has owned a horse will tell you that they are an expensive 'pet' and have amazingly fragile health. Colic comes on suddenly and often strikes an otherwise healthy horse down, costing lots of money no matter what the outcome. Ulcers and cribbing can be a problem, and lameness issues abound. Yet, in Nature, how often do these problems arise? They appear to be related to the unnatural conditions we force horses to live in. Horse owners are finding that a more natural diet and lifestyle helps them keep their animals healthier. While a more natural lifestyle costs more money up front, it can pay for itself in terms of stress and vet bills over the life of the animal.

If you have an animal companion, you can help your pet experience optimal health by giving it appropriate natural living conditions. Since we have bred pets as companions, love is another important aspect of health and happiness for them. A very nice side effect of providing your pets with the most nurturing environment is that it will save you money on vet bills and behavior issues.

∽

Exercise

In order to get the most advantage from Nature, you need to resonate with what it offers. That may mean changing how you think. In this exercise, you will be asked questions about how you regard health. There are no right or wrong answers. You need to be consciously aware of how you think in order to align with natural healing.

1. How much do you feel you are in control of creating the health you desire? You can use a percentage from 0-100% or a number from 0-10.
2. What are you willing to invest in order to experience good health? Money? Time? Effort? A change of mind?

3. Do you believe good health is your natural state, your birthright? Or do you think it is something you have to pay for, struggle to achieve or earn?
4. Do you trust God / the Universe / Nature to provide you with what you need to be healthy? On a 0-10 scale, assign a number, where 0 would mean you have no trust and 10 would mean you have complete trust.
5. Do you feel the earth is a safe and nurturing place to live? You may use a scale of 0-10 to describe how much you agree with that statement.
6. Do you feel that your body and your intuition have a natural intelligence that can be used to guide you toward your goals?

You don't really need to do this exercise to know the answers. You can look at your life experience, and that will tell you what you believe and feel. But by thinking consciously, you can decide if those beliefs or attitudes are helping you to experience what you want or not.

If you are not experiencing the good health you want easily, comfortably and affordably, that can change if you change your attitudes.

2

IS MEDICAL SCIENCE ALWAYS RIGHT?

Scientific "Truth"

Science—the scientific establishment, with a capital 'S'—tends to be rigid in its pronouncements and slow or unwilling to admit error, and while that might not matter a whole lot to you if they reverse their position on the Big Bang, it can have a huge impact on you when they make faulty statements about health topics. One of the most common fallacies these days is that Science knows everything and it knows what is best for you, so you shouldn't question what Science says. Yet as we demonstrated earlier, Science is always discovering new facts, and often those facts lead to a complete reversal of their position.

As an example of how much there is still to learn, take what we are learning about biochemistry. Our knowledge of biochemistry *doubles* every five years. (We have a link in the Resources section to a site which has free posters on biochemical processes. It's way beyond anything you learned in school.) The same is true in all aspects of science, including medical knowledge and its understanding of what creates health and what harms it.

Real science is about the joy of discovery, of adding information to the big picture and tweaking it as needed. Unfortunately, the scientific establishment is not really scientific, in that it abandons the search for knowledge and becomes locked into one paradigm, forgetting that the natural course of science is that of discarding or revising old theories as new facts come to light.

Max Planck, a famous physicist, said,

> A new scientific truth does not triumph by convincing its opponents and making them see the light, but rather because its opponents eventually die, and a new generation grows up that is familiar with it.

By abandoning the search for new knowledge, the scientific establishment abandons science itself, replacing it with arrogance. This is not a modern phenomenon. A few historical examples of medical hubris include:

- The liberal use of opiates, even for babies (19th C)
- The refusal to use sterile procedure during surgery and deliveries of babies (19th C)
- Lobotomies as a solution for mental problems (20th C)
- Mercury as medicine (for thousands of years until the 19th C; still in use by dentists)
- Bloodletting as a cure for illness (for thousands of years until the 19th C)

You're going to ask, didn't anyone object to these horrors? The answer is yes, there are always objectors, but they were marginalized, vilified and ignored (much as they are today). Alfred Russell Wallace, one of the great scientific minds of the 19th century, published a well-researched paper objecting to the practice of vaccination for smallpox, proving it not only wasn't helping, it harmed. Yet the practice continued for many years. Dr. Ignaz

Semmelweis campaigned to get doctors to simply wash their hands between delivering babies, as he had observed that childbed fever that led to many deaths was caused by infection. He was ignored, harassed, lost his job and died in a mental institution. Similar practices continue to this day when a scientist questions medical orthodoxy.

Why does this happen? Scientists are supposed to be seekers of truth. Why wouldn't they be open to new information? Money and power become associated with products and practices, and it becomes very hard to dislodge them. As a result of the slow pace of change, many people are harmed before change occurs. Research is costly and must be funded, and those with the money to fund research often are driven by an agenda other than the search for truth.

All systems are prone to promote bad practices that are later overturned, whether they are religious, economic or social. Think of human sacrifice (religion) and slavery (economics). Once accepted as normal, these practices seem horrific to our 'modern' sensitivities. The problem is that anything can appear normal if it is widely practiced, and it is up to you to decide if that practice fits your values and goals.

It is easy to be shocked by the 'wrong' thinking of hundreds of years ago. But what about some wrong thinking you may have grown up with? Some fairly modern beliefs that have become accepted, but are increasingly being questioned in peer-reviewed studies, include:

- The germ theory of disease, that all microbes are your enemies and should be killed (note the liberal use of antibiotic drugs, antibiotic soaps and chemically-laden hand wipes in grocery stores)
- The sugar/oral hygiene theory of tooth decay
- The theory that vaccination is a safe and effective way to wipe out disease

- Denial that the brain has a lymphatic system, until they 'discovered' it in 2015. (Ayurvedic medicine has known it for thousands of years.)
- The belief that your DNA is your destiny and cannot be changed except via mutation (women removing their breasts because they have certain genes)
- And they still haven't adequately explained the placebo effect, which has wide-ranging implications for health

We must always remember how little we know and avoid arrogance. Galileo said:

> Who would set a limit to the mind of man? Who would dare assert that we know all there is to be known?

In this guide, we will give you the tools for making good decisions about your health when you are presented with all kinds of questionable input from many sources, most of which have an agenda that may not involve you being healthy.

Some of the accepted practices we will ask you to question are vaccinations, GMO foods, the dangers of EMF exposure and the cavalier use of prescription drugs as fixes for various problems. These practices are the bloodletting and lobotomies of our time, and they hold many potential dangers due to not being natural.

Not convinced that a new approach is needed? A study in 2016 by Johns Hopkins showed that medical errors were the number three cause of death in the US at that time. This statistic only relates to reported, confirmed cases of medical error, meaning there are certainly unreported cases as well. Death by doctor is therefore not rare, yet it gets swept under the rug.

A cursory search on google shows that routinely when doctors go on strike, death rates go down. The media won't report that, as it questions the entire basis of our health care system.

These facts are not meant to besmirch the reputations of all doctors; it is just important that you realize the current medical system is fraught with problems of many kinds that impact the health of patients.

From a philosophical point of view, the conventional medical system does not believe in 'cures.' When a disease appears to go away, they term that a 'remission.' This attitude has a greater impact on your health than you might think. It is a clear sign of the foundational belief that medicine is not here to cure you; it is here to mitigate symptoms at best; at worst, its goal is to treat or control those symptoms.

Natural health practitioners, for example, believe Type II diabetes is curable, while conventional doctors do not. Think about how that impacts not only the cost of health care, but your quality of life if you are diagnosed with a disease. We have neighbors who are fairly healthy retirees who have stated to us that they expect to have their health decline and to need long term care before they die. They have accepted the current paradigm being promoted by health care, which has a lot to gain from keeping people alive but in need of drugs and care before they die. Is that the paradigm you want to live by?

We'll be suggesting questions you should ask, new ways to look at these accepted practices and alternative options that could be safer and more effective for your health goals. Finally, there is no way to completely opt out of modern living, but you can mitigate negative side effects if you are aware.

In summary, the scientific method is one of many valid ways of gaining new knowledge, but it is not the only way, nor has it even begun to scratch the surface of all there is to know about human biology. To treat Science as some kind of complete, all-knowing body of information that is infallible is to ignore historical fact, logic and common sense.

Einstein said, "The only thing more dangerous than ignorance is arrogance." We believe that combining the two is a recipe for disaster. Science and technology have intruded on modern living to such an extent that it is hard to get away from the dogma and gadgets and methods, and the pace of change has been so fast without oversight and research to prove long term safety that it behooves you to question, to analyze and to make cautious choices rather than accept advertising and propaganda as your guide to good health.

~

Do You Need Scientific Proof?

> Proof is a dangerous concept. The essence of science is showing that most truth is opinion.
>
> -From "Prayer of the Dragon" by Eliot Pattison

It's good to have facts to back up your opinion. It's just as good to have a strong intuition about the 'rightness' of something. The weakest position is to merely quote some 'authority' instead of thinking for yourself, but we all do that from time to time, because modern life is so busy, there seems to be little time to research, question and inform yourself about most subjects.

It has become the accepted thing to just go along with whichever authority you choose. It might be a person you consider an expert, like your family doctor. It could be a celebrity spokesman, like an actor or athlete you respect or admire. Or possibly you just line up with whatever Science tells you to believe via the media, as in saying if Science hasn't proven it, it can't be so.

You don't need proof to believe something, as most people demonstrate when they quote their favorite authority rather than researching and thinking for themselves. But proof is a wonderful thing. The problem with scientific proof is that science isn't always right, and many studies are faulty in one way or another. Sometimes it's simply the assumptions or experimental design that are off kilter; other times it is more sleazy, like tobacco science that is paid for with a particular agenda in mind.

There is plenty of scientific evidence for many claims being put forward by those who are in favor of a more natural approach to health, but you have to search for it. Thanks to the internet and the ease of independent publishing, there is more information available to you than there was twenty years ago. You just have to sort through it using both your rational mind and your intuition.

Bottom line is make up your own mind about what you believe and ignore those who disagree. If you make decisions based on careful thought, heartfelt intuition and a bit of research, you will be better off by far than those who are blindly following the crowd.

Since we humans know so little about what really creates good health, your opinions may change with time, but they will at least be based on something other than blind faith.

3

HEALTH GOALS & PARADIGMS

What Is Good Health?

What is good health to you? The answer is not as obvious as it might seem. Some people might say good health is not having pain. Others might see it as being able to resolve a bad back. How you perceive health and what your health goals are will impact all your health choices, so it is important to be very clear about them.

Having positive health goals is far better than having negative ones. Wanting to lose weight, to stop arthritis or to get rid of an unwanted symptom is a negative focus. Since what you focus on expands, it is wise to have positive focus on what you want to create instead. (The concept of 'what you focus on expands' goes along with the Law of Attraction and many other metaphysical principles based on 'like attracts like').

Think carefully. What do you want to create in terms of your own physical, mental and emotional health? Some examples of things we include in the concept of good health are:

- Feeling comfortable in your body
- Having plenty of energy for anything you want to do

- Being happy and feeling harmonious
- Having a clear head and being able to remember things well
- Being strong and fit enough to do something in particular
- Enjoying eating meals and feeling comfortable after them

∾

Exercise

Write down your specific, positive health goals and date the document. Now look at them. Are they very specific? Are they truly positive? Do they feel attainable with or without outside assistance? How will you know you have achieved them? How much do you desire to reach those goals, and what are you willing to invest? (You can't expect anything to change if you don't change.)

These are your goals *for now* because your health goals should evolve as life goes on. You will achieve a certain goal and find that you want to set another one. Be patient about the process and keep reminding yourself to visualize what you do want to experience instead of what you are experiencing at this time.

You can have big or small goals. Do what works best for your personality type; don't sabotage yourself by being unreasonable.

Work on trust issues if you feel you have them, meaning trusting that the Universe provides all the support you need, and trusting that you have all the abilities required for success. Work on self-love issues if you have them. Without trust and self-love, it is very hard to make positive changes.

∾

Your Health Paradigm

Now that you have clear health goals, think about how you intend to go about achieving them. For some goals, you won't need any outside help, but for others, you will need to research or consult experts. Which experts will you turn to? Those who resonate with you, who share your basic beliefs, are a good place to start.

Let's look at an example of a goal and how different paradigms would approach achieving it. Say your back constantly gives you pain. You have done what you can and see no improvement. Who will you turn to for help?

In general, a conventional health paradigm focuses on suppressing symptoms as fast as possible without requiring major changes in lifestyle except for life-threatening issues. Drugs and surgery are the main tools, so for your back an allopathic doctor might prescribe muscle relaxants and pain killers and possible surgery to stabilize the spine. The drawbacks of this approach include the side effects of the drugs, especially for long term use, and the success rate of the particular surgery and its risks and side effects.

A holistic approach uses gentler remedies that usually take some time to work and investment on your part, but have fewer side effects and aim at the resolution of root causes. A holistic doctor would probably investigate your medical history and do tests like X-rays to discover the root cause of your back issues, because different issues require different treatment. A series of chiropractic adjustments might resolve a back or neck problem caused by an auto accident. Massage and exercise could strengthen weak muscles that have caused strain leading to pain. If there is bone loss, a new diet that creates stronger bones might be suggested.

Integrative medicine attempts to combine the best of both approaches, but is not really a coherent approach to health as much as an empirical one based on the belief system and experience of the practitioner. A good integrative doctor may, for example, practice conventional medicine but also advocate the use of acupuncture and nutritional remedies at times. For back issues, this professional will present both conventional and holistic options, possibly suggesting you try the holistic ones first, as they are lower risk (if that applies to your situation). Integrative approaches are more empirical (based on what works) than philosophical. This is not to say you should avoid integrative medicine; it may be the best available to you. But be aware that integrative is not philosophically coherent, in that it doesn't fully subscribe to either the conventional or holistic viewpoint.

It is wisest to consult experts who have the same paradigm as you do. If you believe in holistic health and go to a conventional doctor just because it's 'free', but you don't really believe in the conventional approach and even have fear about it, your results won't be good. If you believe in a conventional approach but consult a holistic doctor out of fear, you will likewise not get the results you desire. Perhaps all you care about is results, and you know a good integrative doctor and enjoy working with her.

Work with professionals who are in alignment with your beliefs and attitudes for best results. In other words, don't just do what we or anyone else say; do what you believe is right for you. We explain the importance of beliefs in a later section.

Be willing to change your mind as you move through life pursuing your health goals.

～

Exercise

This exercise will give you an opportunity to consciously think about your beliefs concerning health and how consistent, coherent and helpful they are for helping you achieve good health.

1. How willing are you to regard the process of healing as a journey? Are you impatient and expecting instant results?
2. Do you feel you have all the tools you need to attain these goals? If not, what tools do you lack? Money? Time? Will power? Knowledge?
3. How much are you willing to invest (time, effort and money) to achieve your goals?
4. How can you make up for what you feel you lack? (Example: take a course or read a book in a self-healing technique; quit spending money on cigarettes, junk food and alcohol and save it up to consult with a holistic professional; change your habits and behaviors (eat better, get more sleep)).
5. What health paradigm do you have the most trust in? Conventional medicine? Holistic medicine? Something else? Or are you just following the crowd and have no beliefs?
6. Do you feel there is any benefit to having a coherent viewpoint on health and how to achieve and maintain it? If so, why?
7. Do you consistently consult sources of the type of knowledge you trust and do what they suggest, expecting good results?
8. Has the paradigm you have used in the past given you the results you desire? Are you willing to try something different? Or are you afraid of change or resistant to it?

By taking the time to think about what you believe, you begin to shape outcomes. It doesn't really matter what your answers are, as long as you think carefully and come to heartfelt conclusions. Having a clear point of view and specific goals is required for success.

4
_____

PHYSICAL HEALTH FACTORS

Introduction

Your health is affected by everything your physical body is exposed to in its environment. Think of your body as a closed system within which cells and microorganisms go about the business of keeping you energetic, healthy and happy. That balance can be affected by outside factors, and you have various barriers and systems to mitigate those effects and protect the complex activities that create good health.

Your skin, both that on the outside of your body and that which lines your gut, is the first barrier to environmental toxins and challenges. Yes, the inside of your gut is actually outside of your body, technically speaking.

Interestingly, your gut and outer skin both have microbiota, populations of microorganisms to help maintain the integrity and health of your skin in order to keep it from allowing toxins and dangerous things to enter your body. They also help with the digestive process, allowing the passage of substances you need, in addition to manufacturing vital compounds like serotonin. Without those helpful microorganisms, your skin cannot properly do its duty to protect you, nor can your digestive system provide you with what you need for growth and repair, among other things.

The second layer of protection is your immune system, which is in the cells. There are different types of immunity (we'll discuss that a bit later), and their interrelationship is not completely understood. Medical science in the last hundred or more years has focused mainly on only one aspect of immunity.

Your immune system is vital for good health, yet we know so little about how it functions beyond the basics. When it gets out of whack, you develop autoimmune disease, and that can be very challenging to live with or cure. Autoimmune diseases are on the rise, and traditional medicine is unable to do much to resolve them, which is further evidence that we still have much to learn about how the immune system works. The rise in autoimmune disease may be a result of the increased toxins we are exposed to and deficiencies in diet as well as the high level of stress most people endure. Fortunately, you can make choices to improve your life in all of those areas.

In this section we will examine some of the key external physical factors that affect your body's physical health. What you will learn is that good health is a complex dance modified over many thousands of years by natural factors in the human environment, and understanding how you can alter and improve those factors goes a long way towards helping you reach your health goals.

∽

Food

Let food be thy medicine, and let medicine be thy food

-Hippocrates

While writing this book, I happened to take a stroll down a grocery store aisle that I almost never visit. In fact, it had been literally years since I had browsed the frozen foods aisle of a traditional grocery store which contains meals like TV dinners. (We do the majority of our food shopping at the whole foods store and local farmer's market.) What astonished me was the proliferation of frozen meals for one, meals for families and microwaveable complete dinners. It took both sides of one long aisle to contain what used to take up about a quarter of that space.

This made me aware that fewer and fewer people are preparing meals the natural way. When Nigel was a child in England, his family had a kitchen garden that contained vegetables, herbs and even a few fruit trees, and meals were made or supplemented from the bounty of that plot. When I was a child, I was already generations away from the farm and kitchen gardens. My Mom had been raised in an orphanage and made the same mostly uninspired meals over and over out of mainly canned and frozen ingredients.

Convenience was a key factor to her in meal preparation, as she hated to cook. I remember when instant potato flakes were invented. She quit preparing mashed potatoes from real potatoes, butter and milk because the instant potatoes were much easier. The difference in taste and quality was depressingly obvious even to me as a child. But, unaware of any bad side effects, Mom snatched up anything that meant less time and effort cooking. Powdered orange drink in the form of Tang was invented when I was a child, a space age marvel—drink what the astronauts drink! Marketing was incredibly clever, as it is today, and it sold fake foods as if they were better than the real thing. At the time, we weren't juicing real oranges for breakfast and rarely even had frozen orange juice, but Tang put a stop to even the infrequent use of frozen orange juice concentrate in our home, because it was easier to prepare.

The thrust of this section is to get you thinking about how far from a natural diet you and most modern humans have strayed, and how important it is to become aware of what you are trading for the convenience of things like microwavable dinners and instant drinks and sodas. There is a health price as well as a monetary price for convenience.

These products save time, but they are not natural and often contain artificial preservatives, chemicals and GMO ingredients. They rarely have much food value. And almost none of them are made locally to you. But most importantly, they do not contain the 'information' that makes real, natural food healing, balancing and restorative.

Each geographic location has its own little universe of soil microorganisms that work in conjunction with the microclimate of that area. Man was designed to live in a certain area and eat food from that area that included microorganisms in soil that incorporate vital minerals and other nutrients into the plants, which are passed up the food chain, providing critical elements for good health. Locavores are onto something. Eating food produced locally is good for your health. Grocery store food—even whole foods stores' produce—does not fall into that category. Many of us have not been eating naturally for generations, but we weren't aware that lifestyle choice had a negative impact on health, because the effects are slow and cumulative.

Natural humans eat local food sources in a seasonal fashion, and the human body has adapted to the rhythm of the seasons. In a temperate climate, winter is the season of eating roots, fatty, high protein and hot foods, while spring is traditionally the 'starving' time, when the body is more in tune with spring greens and fewer calories. Modern man eats as if every day is a day of feasting, and so the body never gets to fast or detox and repair; it's always busy digesting food, and unfortunately, most people aren't even eating good food.

Studies of modern hunter-gatherer cultures shows that the gut microbiome—the totality of the microorganisms present in the gut and their genetic material and its effects—changes with the seasonal changes in the food eaten by the hunter-gatherers, and that those shifts allow the body to perform the many complex tasks required to maintain good health. We'll talk more about microbiomes in a later section.

You naturally can tell what food is good for you by using your sense of smell and taste. You can smell and taste when food has spoiled, and that helps you avoid eating it and getting food poisoning. Food that tastes really good is usually good for you, especially if there are no chemical additives like MSG to fool your taste buds.

The exception to that rule is foods high in fats or sugar, because humans are programmed to crave those things, which are rare in Nature, to take advantage of them as much as possible. In our modern society, we are so rich that we have many opportunities to eat fatty and sweet foods, natural and fake, and people tend to binge on them. Processed sugar has been shown to be highly addictive, which isn't surprising given our genetic propensity to love sweet foods like honey. So while taste is a good indicator in general of what is healthy, you have to take into account our genetic tendency towards craving fats and sugar and factor that into your food choices by choosing natural sources of these things and eating them in moderation.

However, in general, your taste buds won't lead you wrong. You almost certainly can tell the difference between mashed potatoes made from your garden using organic milk and butter, from mashed potatoes made from instant flakes and using margarine and powdered milk. I know for certain you can tell the difference between a home-grown tomato and one bought in a grocery store, just by the look, feel and taste. You are kidding yourself if you think that 'all the natural goodness' of real food can be duplicated in a lab or with chemicals. Your sense of taste knows, and it tries to tell you.

In addition to eating high quality food, how you eat matters. Eating should be a joyful and enjoyable experience, not just a quick way to refuel. Modern humans spend as little time as possible preparing food and bolt their meals down, often watching TV or their cell phones at the same time. Scientific studies now have shown that eating with intention, having a ritual of some kind, contributes to improved taste and enjoyment, but also a strengthening of the gut microbiome and tantalizingly, possibly improves genetic expression.

Food is fuel, but it is much more. We need to start seeing food not as simply fuel for the body, as if the body is a machine, but as an integral part of our being able to experience well-being and interact well with our environment. Sayer Ji, founder of GreenMedInfo, says,

> We have crossed a critical threshold in the past few decades where food can no longer be considered simply as a source of caloric content, minerals and vitamins, and building blocks for the body-machine... Rather, food carries very specific forms of biologically meaningful information (literally 'to put form into'), without which our genetic and epigenetic infrastructure cannot function according to its intelligent design.

One example of this: Small vesicles called exosomes and exosome-like nanoparticles have been discovered in plants and animals, and early research demonstrates that these are at least one of the carriers of information between the food you eat and your body. Activities like fighting inflammation and modifying gene expression have been shown to be part of the job of plant exosomes, and it is postulated that they may help explain why certain foods are so healing and healthy. This is breaking research, tapping into that unknown body of knowledge we refer to, and it supports the contention that natural is good for you.

The research indicates that unprocessed food is healthier, and that plants have healing properties. Does this mean you should turn to a purely plant-based diet? No. Humans in nature were designed to be omnivores—just check out our dentition—and restricting your diet to only plants leads to potentially serious vitamin deficiencies. You certainly don't need as much animal protein as most modern humans ingest, and you should vary your meat intake to include more than just muscle meat or one type of meat protein, because organs like liver and kidney, when they are clean, are wonderful sources of nutrition. In Nature, humans probably ate a diet that was mostly plant-based, but also included animal and insect protein sources.

Some people choose a vegetarian diet for ethical reasons rather than scientific or nutritional ones, and if that is your choice, be careful to supplement what you are missing out on. But don't feel superior to carnivores, because recent studies show that plants have consciousness and intelligence and are able to communicate, and once you realize that, feasting on plants instead of animals becomes a bit hypocritical. The up side of this revelation, which many of us believed after reading *The Secret Life Of Plants* in the 1970s, is that science is finally establishing that there is a consciousness in all beings, animals and plants, that consciousness exists even in rocks, and eventually, research will probably support the long-held ancient belief of the interconnection of all life.

So are there any valid ethical concerns in terms of the food you eat? Yes. The so-called ethical issues overlap with practical, scientific ones, and it is important to point them out to you. The plants and animals you use as food are not identical to what humans in the wild eat. Hunter-gatherers eat wild plants and animals or the occasional carcass left by other predators. When humans began practicing agriculture, some 10,000 years ago—and that is recent in terms of human biological history—they began to modify plants and animals to make it easier to raise them for food.

The minute species began to be selectively bred for certain traits, like size, docility and ease of feeding or fast growth rates, Nature's design was altered. In most cases, their lifestyle was also altered. Fast forward to the past hundred or so years. Since World War II, agribusiness has taken over from small family farms in the US. Their goal is simple: put out as much food as possible with as little investment as possible. Agribusiness relies on consumers believing an egg is an egg, and corn is corn. Most people don't realize that raising animals in crowded conditions and feeding them cheap food causes stress and disease which then affects the food quality for the consumer. And yet, at the same time, most of us hate grocery-store tomatoes and long for home grown, so we do have an intuitive awareness of the lack of quality. Plants grown on depleted soil lack minerals, lack flavor and lack nutrition. But beyond taste, most people are ignorant about how the living conditions of food animals and plants ultimately affect not only the animal's health and quality of life, but their value to you as food.

Raising plants and animals for food in as natural a condition as possible is expensive compared to factory farming, but it pays off in giving good quality food packed with nutrients. In a sense, agribusiness creates negative food karma. Buying from companies that are humane and provide natural growing and living conditions pays you back with high quality food and good karma. Once again, natural is best.

But once you have your ingredients, whatever they are, you can perform a critical function that will enhance the healthiness of your food. If you fail to serve food with love and gratitude, or you don't enjoy eating your meal, you are missing out on many of the benefits of eating, and that leads to ill health. Studies show that eating slowly and making meals a happy ritual enhances the value of the food you eat.

Once you ingest food, it is vital to digest it well. (We'll talk about the gut microbiome in a later section; it is absolutely vital to your health.) Local, pesticide-free, non-GMO, unprocessed foods are not only rich in vitamins and minerals. They contain gut microorganisms and enzymes and genetic elements that science has yet to discover that are not present in processed foods. They 'feed' you.

Obesity is a complex issue that is rampant in modern society, but at least in part it is tied to the fact that a poor diet leads to unbalanced hormones and cravings. Your body knows what it lacks, and it will keep seeking those things. You can eat all the Cheetos, candy bars and chips you want, and you will not be healthy; you will just get fat. Plus, you will always be hungry, because the body craves minerals and other needed nutrients you cannot get in fast food and junk food, and it will try to keep you eating, because you are programmed to eat until you satisfy the needs of your body. We are literally starving to death amid plenty; the excess weight just hides that fact.

We are only beginning to discover the many factors affecting nutrition that Science never suspected, but those discoveries point to eating as being far more than just shoving calories into your body if you want optimal health and longevity. In fact, recent discoveries show that much ancient wisdom about health is spot on.

In an ideal world, we would all have gardens where we grew a lot of our food, and we would also feed the soil organisms carefully and be sure we did everything organically. We would eat unprocessed foods seasonally and make mealtimes calm and joyful.

Reverting to that lifestyle, of course, subjects you to the vagaries of weather and other factors which affect crop yield. Also, if you tried to grow your own food, it would be a massive challenge to produce the diverse array of species required for an optimal diet, as well as take more time and energy than most people feel they have. There are many challenges to creating a more natural diet, and it will probably be necessary to compromise. We aren't suggesting you have to become a farmer to enjoy good health, but your health will improve the closer you get to a natural model in terms of what you eat.

How many steps removed from this lifestyle are you? Probably a few generations. But don't worry. You can improve your situation, no matter what you are now doing. Do the exercises to get an idea where you can become more natural in your diet.

~

Exercise #1

A. How would you describe the difference in taste between:

- A home grown tomato and a store-bought one
- Water from a mountain stream as opposed to tap water

Granted, if you don't have the opportunity to sample one or both of the above, you may need to substitute something else, like farmed salmon versus wild caught or tap water versus bottled. Use your own experience to come up with some things you can compare.

What descriptive words and phrases did you use? You can tell the difference. Your sense of taste is meant to help you choose food that is full of nutrition, life force and all the things you need to thrive. If you use your taste buds as nature intended, and if you choose food that tastes better, meaning more alive, you will be using your senses as Nature intended.

An interesting side note is that grocery stores years ago began to substitute large and unblemished for nutritious and healthy produce. Nutritious and healthy produce isn't always blemish-free, and often may be smaller than what you buy in the grocery store. Size and cosmetic appearance are not a substitute for true food value, but you may have to overcome your natural tendency to judge in order to make changes in your buying habits.

Remember: the tendency to love sweets and fatty foods is also programmed into your body, because these are good for you if they are natural and in the right amounts at the right times. Those types of foods are relatively rare in Nature, and we are programmed to binge on them.

Natural sweets like honey are actually healthy in moderation, but there are few of them. Even maple syrup and molasses are processed sweets, but they are superior to high fructose corn syrup. Humans now produce fake sweets and bad fatty foods that contribute to disease by appealing to those natural tastes. So not only do you need to eat natural foods that taste good; you need to eat them in the right proportion, amount, and in the right season for your body to thrive.

B. What is your attitude about food, eating and nutrition? Do you sit down and enjoy a meal with loved ones, or do you rush and eat whatever is easiest as if eating is just another chore to tick off your list? How you eat and regard food, your relationship with food, is an expression of your beliefs.

The healthiest attitude is one of enjoying good food, knowing it is helpful to you, loving good tastes and eating slowly and with gusto. If you don't have that outlook, cultivating it is a very good first step towards a healthier life.

For many people, food is the enemy, as they have developed food allergies. Address that attitude if you want to see change. Food allergies are a sign of an imbalanced immune system and poor digestion, as well as suggestive of liver or histamine issues. They prevent you from developing a positive attitude about food and nourishment.

C. What differences could there be between flour tortillas handmade by your Mom from organic flour and those bought at the grocery store that are produced in a factory situation? Try to think of at least 3 differences.

∿

Exercise #2

The following questions are designed to let you see how far you have departed from the diet Nature intended you to eat.

1. What percentage of your intake of liquids is pure (not tap) water?
2. Do you drink caffeinated or alcoholic beverages or soda?
3. What percent of the food you eat is organic?
4. Do you have an organic garden of any type?
5. Do you buy at the local Farmer's Market often?
6. What percentage of your food is readymade, as in frozen foods, bought bakery goods and canned goods?
7. How much microwaving of food do you do?
8. Do you feed your pets a raw food diet?
9. What percentage of your pets' diet is processed food, like dry or canned, and where do you buy it (grocery store/pet store/whole foods store)?
10. Do you feed your pets tap water or filtered water?
11. How much snacking do you do?
12. How often do you dine out?
13. Do you use money and time as excuses not to cook or buy organic ingredients?

∼

Water

Water is required for life. Most people are aware that the human body is made up mostly of water, but scientists in the past gave water a passive role, that of a solvent for things like proteins or a carrier, as with blood cells. While dehydration was known to be 'bad' for you and drinking enough water was always advised, there was not much information and few theories of why water is so important to good health.

In the latter part of the twentieth century and onwards, groundbreaking theories were put forward stating that water is far more important for health and does far more interesting things that we previously thought. But putting that awareness into practice—that just hasn't happened yet.

It is those new theories about water's importance that lead to suggestions by holistic healers to be sure to drink plenty of pure water every day. F. Batmanghelidj, M.D. (Dr. Batman for short) went so far as to postulate and present anecdotal evidence that chronic dehydration is the cause of many common diseases in today's world, from stomach pain to back problems. Our culture's tendency to drink anything but water has led to terrible health problems that in many cases could be avoided if people drank enough water, but they have been seduced into drinking coffee, alcoholic beverages and soda instead, and those liquids do not equal water.

In *The Fourth Phase Of Water*, Gerald Pollack postulates that water is more than just a solvent in your cells. In living systems and sometimes in Nature, water appears in a phase that is not like a solid, liquid or gas. This fourth phase has electrical properties that help drive the processes that take place in your body. While Dr. Batman theorized that many disease symptoms are born of chronic dehydration, Pollock has taken it a step further and shows the vital importance of having enough water in the proper form to stay healthy. He mentions that nonnative EMFs (electromagnetic fields) negatively affect this unique structure of water. We'll be talking about EMFs in a later chapter.

There is so much we just don't know about how your body uses water, but we are getting tantalizing hints that it is way more important than we realized—just as we are with food.

A further development in our understanding of water came from Dr. Emoto's work that showed water responds to intention and emotions directed at it, changing its form in ways that show clearly in photomicrographs. Water therefore interacts with human intelligence, and perhaps also interacts with other types of intelligence; water, like food, carries information. The implications of this research are that we as humans can alter the structure and energies of things around us. The story of Jesus changing water to wine in the Bible comes to mind.

Intention is indeed very powerful, and we should consciously harness that for our health goals. The use of intention is a skill, and most people are not masterful at using it without training, but it is worthwhile to start using intention to consciously show your commitment to your goals.

Being aware that pure water (not tap water) in proper amounts is vital for health is a priceless bit of knowledge that could help you avoid being diagnosed with diseases that are simply signs of dehydration.

Do the exercise and think about how you are interacting with water and using it for your health.

~

Exercise

1. How much water do you drink daily?
2. Do you drink filtered water, tap water, bottled water, spring water or well water?

~

Microbiomes

Your skin is your first and most important layer of protection from harmful elements in your environment. It turns away the bad and uses the good, and it does so mostly with the help of microorganisms that live on and in you. It is vital that you protect the balance of the complex activities of these microorganisms to maintain good health.

In our culture, we damage or kill off our skin microbiota—the term that relates to yeast, bacteria, fungi and viruses that dwell on and in you—by using personal care products with chemicals. Soaps, antibiotics, shampoos, hair dyes, makeup and suntan lotion provide challenges to your skin microbiota. Such products (other than soap and simple makeup) didn't even exist a hundred years ago. If you use any personal care products, be sure they do not have antibiotic properties, nor chemicals of any type.

It's hard to find truly natural products, meaning products with natural, healthful ingredients, but it is worth the effort. Your skin absorbs toxins, leading to pressure on liver and kidney function. By reducing toxic load, you improve health. You'll also save money that can be put to use buying good, organic food. And you will reduce your chances of some kinds of cancer, because many toxins have been shown to be carcinogenic.

Most people are aware that the skin is your largest organ. They think of the skin as that outer body covering. But there is another, equally important skin layer that is protecting you from the external environment: your gut lining. The inside of your gut, from mouth to anus, is actually outside of your body. And its surface area is approximately 100 times larger than your outer skin.

All of your skin has a microbiome, a totality of microorganisms and their genetic material that dwell there and perform vital health functions. The location and function determines the composition of the microbiome. Your outer skin will have far different microorganisms than your gut. All of these microorganisms are 'good' bacteria.

The old 'Germ Theory' of disease, which a Google search will tell you is the accepted theory of disease at this time, began in the 1800s. The core of this theory was that bacteria and other microorganisms are responsible for all illness; therefore, they are bad for you. My parents grew up in the early 20th Century, and they were programmed to be afraid of bacteria, because they had been told they cause disease and infection, which were serious threats to life when they were young.

This theory is incomplete at the very least, and just plain wrong at the worst. Demonizing microorganisms has created a mindset of us vs. them. Antibiotic drugs were therefore welcomed as miracles, and from there, it was a short drive to developing antibacterial soaps, wipes and all kinds of other things to kill those nasty critters, including chlorinated water.

The reality is this: 99% of metabolic processes are supported, coded for or organized by bacterial and viral DNA, not human DNA. Our health is actually totally dependent on microbes and their DNA. Microorganisms are vital for health. You can't live without them. They determine not only your digestive health, but your mental function and emotional state.

In recent years, a weak attempt has been made to rectify this outlook by characterizing some bacteria as 'good.' The average person is aware that probiotics have 'good' bacteria that help digestion, but the reality of our dependence on our microbiota is glossed over and not fully understood, so there is still an overuse of antibiotics and antibiotic products. These practices are becoming serious global threats to human health, as in the case of new super strains of bacteria that have evolved as a response to this practice.

Conventional medicine knows beyond a shadow of a doubt that antibiotic abuse is responsible for creating super-bacteria, yet in many, if not most, cases, if you go to a clinic with what sounds like an infection, you will be given antibiotics without being tested to see if bacteria are the cause of your problem. Not only does this breed stronger 'bad' guys; it kills off all the 'good' bacteria, which in a sense is worse. How many doctors give you instructions for restoring your gut bacteria after antibiotic use? And even if they do, it is probably restricted to 'take a probiotic.'

Your microbiome, the totality of the organisms living in and on you plus their genetic input, on which you depend for health, is very complex and responds not only to food—we've talked about the importance of eating real food—but to environmental factors as well, such as EMFs (electromagnetic fields) and geopathic stress.

You cannot support a complex living ecosystem on fake foods that have no biological information. If used as replacements for 'real' food, Cheetos and donuts and Diet Coke are a death sentence to your health, because they lack any of the vital and important factors that contribute to good health.

Another factor to consider is that your gut is your 'second brain' and communicates with your brain via the vagus nerve to coordinate many functions, from digestion to emotional health and intuition. If your gut is not balanced and healthy, if it lacks good gut microbiota, your second brain cannot function well, and many functions will be disturbed.

Your vagus nerve is the longest cranial nerve, and it wanders through the body, ultimately connecting both brains. Studies have shown that the vagus mostly sends messages back to the brain from the various organs it visits, rather than the other way around. The vagus nerve plays such a key role in so many aspects of health that it behooves you to keep your vagus nerve balanced and healthy. Many people suffer from an imbalance of the vagus nerve, leading to a number of unpleasant symptoms. You can easily google vagus nerve symptoms, and you will see they are many and varied. Some mimic serious health conditions. Restoring the tone of the vagus nerve is important, and studies show that deep breathing, toning and reducing stress are all ways to achieve that.

If you want to be healthy, the first thing you must do is support your microbiota, make sure they are strong, diverse and balanced. Ayurveda, the ancient Indian system of medicine, teaches that 85% of ill health begins in the gut, and we believe this is true. If you care for your gut and its microbiota, you will resolve many health problems.

The following exercise gives you a chance to think about how your behaviors affect your microbiomes and thus, your health.

∽

Exercise

1. Have you ever taken antibiotics? How often have you taken a probiotic supplement afterwards?
2. Do you shower in chlorinated (tap) water or drink it?
3. Do you use personal care products like shampoo, hair dye and skin lotion that have any manmade ingredients?
4. Do you eat fermented foods? How often?
5. Do you eat a lot of processed foods (frozen pizza, junk food, frozen meals)?
6. Do you suffer from poor digestion or food and skin allergies?

∽

Supplements

It doesn't really matter how or where you live. You are probably going to have some nutritional deficiencies. It isn't only poor people who suffer because they don't have the means to purchase good food; rich people historically have also suffered from deficiencies and imbalances, just different ones from poor folks.

Modern humans are essentially rich people who are spending money on nutritionally deficient and even toxic foods, and they are suffering from a lot of deficiencies as a result. Most Americans are deficient in magnesium, vitamin D, vitamin K2 and various B vitamins. The way to remedy this problem is to eat good quality food. But even the best modern diet is going to have some deficiencies.

Nutritional supplements are useful as a short term remedy for deficiencies in the diet. They are usually manmade substances designed using limited knowledge of nutrition and sometimes have additives and binders that lead to allergic reactions. Bioavailability—the ease of assimilation—varies a lot, and in fact, poor quality supplements just pass through your body or are treated as toxins.

Supplements are not a panacea or a substitute for proper eating choices. However, periodically, you will probably need to supplement certain vitamins and minerals to obtain optimal health.

You are unique, so there is no laundry list we can give you that will be perfect, but as knowledge of nutrition grows, there will be further developments that help you create a better balance. It will probably be many years before a true and full understanding is available (if it ever is), so be cautious and use supplements mostly short term and with caution, because what is recommended as absolutely necessary now will probably be found to be harmful in the future. Case in point: antioxidants. For years, antioxidants were pushed as a necessary part of a healthy program. Get rid of free radicals! Now, it has been shown that a certain amount of free radicals are required for good health. Oh dear! This is just one example of how things can be expected to change dramatically over time as new knowledge is discovered.

There are some supplements that are vital for good health, and depending on your diet, you could benefit from periodic supplementation. This is an example of where dowsing is helpful so you don't waste money. If you are an accurate dowser, you can dowse how deficient you are, how well a certain brand of supplement will work and whether there will be negative side effects. Otherwise, you just go with your intuition. It is helpful if you have some understanding of what each vitamin or mineral does, but always bear in mind, there is so much we don't know.

Here are some supplements worth considering, because modern humans often are deficient in them:

- Trace minerals
- Magnesium
- B vitamins as a complex
- Vitamin C
- Probiotic supplements after antibiotic use or any insult to the digestive tract
- Concentrated butter oil/fermented cod liver oil

The last supplement is actually a natural artisan food made of concentrated butter oil and fermented cod liver oil, rather than a lab formula like most supplements. It has been shown to be a decent replacement for foods that give you K2 and other fat soluble vitamins required for good health. Modern humans don't eat those foods anymore, and dental issues, the need for orthodontics, and increased heart disease, Alzheimer's, obesity and cancer result from the deficiencies. We use this particular supplement daily. There is a link in the Resources section to a good source. Until we get more information, we will continue to supplement this one to replace missing foods in our diet. It can be considered more of an artisan food than a supplement in terms of ingredients. Thus, it is in alignment with our goal not to take manmade supplements too often.

Supplements can be a useful part of a healthy diet, but you need to exercise good judgment and intuition to avoid negative outcomes and wasted money.

In general, if you feel you have deficiencies, and you aren't well-read in nutrition, it is wisest to take a good quality 'complete' vitamin and mineral supplement for a period of time and then evaluate your health, rather than supplementing just one mineral or vitamin. It is too easy to create imbalance when you only take one mineral, because often, they work in pairs. Calcium and magnesium work together, for example, as do zinc and copper. By loading one of the pair, you can create an imbalance in the other. Taking a balanced complete supplement is a good first step for resolving deficiencies.

∼

Exercise

The following questions will help you evaluate your stand on supplementation and decide if you want to make any changes. Remember, we still have such an incomplete understanding about proper nutrition that you want to stay open to new ideas.

1. Do you take nutritional supplements? How often?
2. Do you research for the most bioavailable brand and formula?
3. How much money are you spending on supplements?
4. Do you see results with supplements?
5. Have you ever seen side effects that were unwanted when you took a supplement?
6. Do you use supplements as a substitute for a proper diet or to shore up the occasional deficiency?
7. When you have symptoms, do you look online to see if they might be caused by a nutritional deficiency?

∼

Toxins

All environments have toxins, substances which are poisonous to you. You can't escape the fact that some things support good health, while others don't. Being aware of toxins and how to deal with them helps you to create optimal health and reach your health goals.

Your liver is your major detoxification organ, but toxins can affect all parts of your body. Avoiding them is a major health strategy; detoxification is another. Each approach has its place in your health regimen.

Naturally occurring toxins would include arsenic in your well water and ash and gases from a volcano polluting your air. There are toxins in the food you eat. Some are natural, while others are manmade. The natural toxins mostly have developed as ways to keep animals from eating plants or to keep animals from preying on other animals. For example, milkweed, like many plants, uses toxic substances called alkaloids to discourage those who would eat it, and to a great extent, it is a successful strategy, but one insect in particular has developed the ability to eat milkweed with impunity. The alkaloids in milkweed plants are incorporated into the body of Monarch butterfly caterpillars when they eat the plant. The toxic chemicals end up stored in the wings of the adult, and the alkaloids make birds sick if they eat the butterfly. The insect has developed a way of using the toxins so it can continue to eat the plant unaffected; in fact, it uses the alkaloids as its own defense. Ideally for the plant, the toxin would repel the creature eating it, but the coevolution of species allows all kinds of adaptations to take place.

Many of the foods we eat, the reproductive parts of plants in particular (fruits, seeds and nuts) often contain substances that are irritating or poisonous to animals who eat them. Grains (which are a type of grass seed), beans and nuts have lectins to discourage ingestion by animals, and those lectins have been shown to lead to leaky gut syndrome, among other things. The controversy about removing grain or gluten from the diet rages on, and until we know more about how grains affect digestion, we won't be able to pinpoint the exact reason a grain-free diet helps so many people, but probably lectins are a major culprit. Regardless, most people benefit from removing or seriously limiting grains in their diets.

The nightshade family, which includes tomatoes, potatoes, peppers and eggplants, all have toxic substances in their vegetative (green) parts. For a long time, people avoided eating nightshades because they knew that parts of them were toxic. Some people react to the fruits of nightshades with joint pain, but the fruits are far less toxic than the green parts of the plant.

Bottom line, plants want to make other plants, not feed you or me, and so the reproductive parts of plants often have toxic substances. Is there any way around it? By germinating seeds, you neutralize the effects of the lectins, and that is one reason sprouting is so popular. Another example: soaking almonds is often used as a way to limit the negative effects of ingesting nuts. In a sense, by mimicking the natural process of seed germination or actually starting it, you activate changes in the chemical structure of the seed or nut which makes ingestion safer and even nutritious.

So Nature has plenty of examples of natural toxins in the food you eat and the water you drink. Man has added far more toxins with the use of pesticides, behaviors that pollute soil, water, air and food and the use of preservatives and other chemicals. Additionally, heavy metal exposure via dental work, vaccines, polluted water and cooking or eating implements create toxic situations. Lead was once used in cosmetics, and in modern times, we accept the use of cosmetics that contain lots of chemicals.

Spraying in the skies has become prevalent in the last decade or two, but governments don't own up to it. The materials in the aerosols contain toxins that are showing up in snow on mountaintops, leading to concerns not only for inhaled allergies and toxicity, but contamination of soil and water.

Pharmaceutical medicines are formulated to help people, but often have toxic side effects on liver and kidneys, because they are not natural substances the body can easily break down. Drugs and breakdown products of pharmaceuticals are becoming prevalent in city water, as it is not treated to remove them.

How many of these manmade toxins were prevalent two hundred years ago? Very few. The Industrial Revolution and the modern age have ushered in the commonplace use of chemicals, the practice of pollution and with them, an increase in toxicity.

An amazing amount of 'normal living' involves exposure to toxins. Do the exercise and give some thought to ways you are exposed to manmade toxins.

~

Exercise

1. Do you have mercury amalgam dental fillings?
2. Do you eat only organic, non-GMO foods?
3. Do you use personal care products or pharmaceuticals?
4. Do you cook with aluminum pans or teflon-coated pans?
5. Do you live in a city?

~

Body Harmony

Your body was designed to move. Modern man lives a largely sedentary lifestyle, sitting at desks all day, commuting to and from work in cars and subways, lounging on the couch in evenings. When you combine this sedentary lifestyle with poor nutrition, you get structural challenges like bad backs, creaky joints and obesity, among other things.

Lymphatic drainage is a vital part of your body's detoxification process, and it works best if your body is in motion. Walking is the most natural form of exercise, yet modern humans have done everything they can to eliminate walking. Historically, rich people rode horses and in wagons and carriages to avoid the time and effort of walking as a means of travel. Now, we use cars, trains and planes.

How you hold your body is another factor in health. Having poor habits in feeding and exercising your body leads to weak muscles and poor posture, which leads to pain and decreased functionality.

If your lifestyle doesn't give you time to move your body and hold it naturally, you will need to find ways to compensate for that in order to experience good health. We'll talk about options in the chapter on taking action.

∼

Sleep

Sleep is required for health, but in spite of many years of research, much remains unknown about the restorative powers of sleep. Sleep deprivation is a popular form of torture, and unfortunately, modern humans often deprive themselves of sleep, turning to sugar, coffee and drugs to give them a boost to get through the day on less than adequate sleep. But there is no substitute for a good night's sleep, so it is important you make time for your body to get the rest it needs.

It has long been known that sleep is restorative, but there are probably other benefits yet to be discovered. Take as an example the glymphatic system. In 2015, it was discovered that the brain has its own lymphatics, the glymphatic system. Proper lymphatic drainage is vital for health, and it is possible this activity in the brain, which only takes place while you sleep, is one reason sleep-deprived people do not function well. The glymphatic system removes on average three pounds of toxins a year from the brain, and if the glymphatic system isn't operating well, those toxins will build up, leading to dis-ease.

Sleep is dependent on the hormone melatonin, which is regulated by natural day and night light cycles, called circadian rhythms. We will

discuss in a later chapter the habits and technological innovations
that have contributed to messed up circadian rhythms, making it
even harder to sleep.

∾

Light

Sunlight is a natural form of electromagnetic radiation that humans,
and indeed all species on earth, have evolved to take advantage of.
Sunlight is used by plants to make food. We eat plants and benefit
from the conversion of electromagnetic energy to starches and
carbohydrates. But our interaction with the sun goes way beyond
that. Our bodies respond to light and dark, creating what are called
circadian rhythms that control all the processes in our bodies. When
those rhythms are disturbed, dis-ease is sure to follow.

People who live at high latitudes (closer to the North or South Poles
than the equator) can have health challenges related to being
deprived of sunlight. One well-documented one is the inability to
make enough vitamin D if you live in high latitudes, although, since
we do not know all there is to know about human biology, there may
well be compensatory systems available to those living at higher
latitudes, as the Inuit seem to have adapted well to very challenging
and unusual living conditions in high northern latitudes. At this
time, we don't know what has made it possible for them to stay
healthy in the low light environment. Discovering that would be
useful in helping people living in far northern and far southern
hemisphere climates.

Many decades ago, Science recognized SAD, seasonal affective
disorder, as a condition caused by not getting enough sunlight,
which leads to depression.

We are living in exciting times, where new discoveries happen every
year, showing how connected and attuned we are to our natural

environment, and what price we pay when we disturb that balance. As we discover more about the important role of natural EMFs like sunlight and the function of our bodies via biophotons and the altered state of water, we can begin to see how vital the right types of light / EMFs are and how disruptive unnatural ones can be to our health.

In a later chapter, we will talk about technology and how it has caused problems via non-native EMFs and blue light. We are only beginning to understand how important it is to get out in the sun and avoid manmade EMFs and blue light.

___

5

MENTAL, EMOTIONAL & ENERGETIC HEALTH FACTORS

Everything is mind over matter. Every disease is mental first.
Everything is about thought. Everything is about vibration.
Everything is about the way you feel. Practice scenarios that feel
good—and never mind reality. Reality is only a brief moment in time
that you keep repeating.

Abraham-Hicks

Introduction

In the previous chapter, we examined physical factors that affect the
health of your body; in this chapter, we will look at factors that are
just as powerful, but often are ignored because they are invisible or
have not been accepted by modern culture as having an effect on
health. Most of these factors cannot yet be measured using scientific
instruments, but ancient medical systems and anecdotal evidence of
their existence and effects are compelling.

This chapter will touch on some of the more commonly accepted
energetic health factors. Bear in mind that we still know very little
about all aspects of energetic health. Scientific studies are showing
more and more that ancient wisdom is correct about the many and

complex factors that affect health, including invisible ones like energy, making it reasonable to examine and use those systems.

Many ancient cultures preach that all health begins in a nonphysical aspect of the human, what is often called the subtle energy body. Oriental and Indian cultures for thousands of years have acknowledged the existence of energetic aspects of the human being, and the medical practices of those cultures use this knowledge to help cure illness and create better health.

In those traditions, it is consistently believed that poor health originates in the energy body first, and if untreated, it eventually manifests in the physical body. If this is true, then we need to pay greater attention to the health and well-being of our subtle energy body, because in so doing, we foster better physical health.

This chapter will examine some of the key energetic factors that lead to imbalances that eventually cause ill health. In a later chapter, we will suggest some action you can take to have a healthier subtle energy body.

∾

Beliefs

> Whether you believe you can do a thing or not, you are right.

-Henry Ford

It is becoming popular in the spiritual and natural health community to talk about the power of beliefs, but it seems there are no quick fixes for eradicating faulty ones, and that leads even the most fervent 'believer' frustrated.

Possibly, this frustration is common because people don't understand the concept of how the subconscious affects our experience of reality. They think of beliefs as what you consciously want or think is true. They don't grasp the fact that the real definition of a belief relates to your vibrational frequency, the energy tone you are broadcasting with no conscious effort. They don't understand that your vibration is largely dependent on your subconscious.

Your subconscious is running your life almost all the time, so you must pay attention to what it believes, and the shocking truth is, most of the time it is in direct opposition to what you consciously want, and guess which wins? The subconscious does, because it is in charge of survival.

All those affirmations you say? Pretty pointless in most cases. Affirmations are you trying to override your subconscious with conscious thoughts, and that is not very effective for most people.

So where do beliefs come in for your health, and what can you do about them? First, you need to become aware of the subconscious programming you have that may be impacting your health negatively. Here are some examples of subconscious beliefs, both good and bad, that you may have that will impact your health process. If you consciously believe them as well, they can be very powerful for good or bad.

- You are stupid; you are not powerful; others know best
- You are a victim of things you cannot control
- Health is costly
- Good health is not your birthright; health is something you must work at
- Your DNA is your destiny
- Your body has the ability to heal itself
- You don't need to be an MD to know how to be healthy
- You have to have a doctor tell you how to be healthy
- You need a college degree to understand health
- Your intuition can guide you in health choices
- Disease is caused by germs

- You're going to have a long, downhill slide and then die
- Getting healthy is hard

In reading this list, you are aware which beliefs you consciously agree with, but you cannot know which ones you subconsciously agree with, because the definition of subconscious is 'below the conscious' level, meaning you don't know what goes on there. So how do you figure out what your subconscious believes? A good dowser can dowse which beliefs are active at the subconscious level, but most people are not accurate dowsers. Fear not! Another way of determining what your subconscious believes is to look around you. What happens to you, what your experience is, is a sign of what your subconscious expects and believes, as opposed to what you consciously desire.

For example, if you are spending a ton of money on health, your subconscious believes health is costly. If you don't feel competent to help yourself be healthy, you have one or more of the related beliefs in the list. If you do what your doctor says even when it feels wrong, you lack belief in yourself and your intuition.

There are various methods that can shift the energy of faulty subconscious beliefs, but the easiest one is to become aware that you have a faulty belief; to decide you don't want to have it; to substitute a better belief; to take action to show your intent.

A broad, longstanding belief is harder to shift than a recent, small one. Start with those you consciously want to change rather than trying to shift a belief you consciously believe is correct, or self-sabotage will cause you to get stuck

The placebo effect is an example of beliefs at work. A certain percentage of people receiving a sugar pill instead of medicine get well. This is because the drug isn't the solution; a change of mind is the best medicine. If you believe something will work at all levels of your being, it works. Note: Consciously believing isn't enough, or faith healing would work for everyone.

Become aware of what your subconscious beliefs are by how you feel, think about and experience health, and then take action to shift beliefs that aren't working for you. We'll have some suggestions in a later chapter.

～

Trauma & Emotions

As with beliefs, what you feel matters when your goal is to create good health. Trauma and so-called 'negative' emotions are counterproductive to being healthy. Remember the axiom that 'like attracts like' and what you focus on expands, and you can understand why trauma or fear, anxiety and sadness can impact your health negatively.

Dr. Ryke Geerd Hamer, a surgeon, has shown that in many cases, cancer begins some years (often within two) after an unresolved conflict, the ongoing negative emotions having an effect on a particular organ or area of the body, which leads to the development of cancer. He speculates that adrenalin exhaustion, vitamin C and niacin depletion/deficiency and immune system suppression are involved.

I can give anecdotal support of his theory from my own family. My mother's favorite among the three of us girls was my youngest sister. She and my mother did not have a close relationship, but my mother doted on her, and their interactions were fairly upbeat on the surface until something happened one day. My 87-year-old mother was having some dementia by then, and she couldn't tell me why my sister had declared that she wouldn't ever speak to her again. Since my sister was also not speaking to me, I had no way of helping Mom resolve the crisis. She was deeply injured at my sister's behavior, but nothing she did repaired the damage; my sister continued to refuse to see or talk to Mom. Less than one year after this event, my mother was diagnosed with lung cancer. She had never smoked in her life, nor had she been exposed to known lung carcinogens of any kind. In Oriental medicine, the lung is the seat of grief or loss; those were emotions my Mom was experiencing deeply. She died less than six months after the diagnosis. There is no doubt in my mind that the emotional trauma triggered the manifestation of lung cancer, just as Dr. Hamer suggests.

But what is really mind-blowing is that it isn't just present life trauma that undermines health; even trauma experienced by your ancestors can negatively affect your health and indeed, your life experience in general. Epigenetics studies support this contention.

The term epigenetics emerged in the 1990s with variable meanings, but in general it reflects a new understanding about how incredibly flexible your genome is; that genes can be turned on or off by many factors. What this means is that your genes are not your destiny. The old Nature vs. Nurture argument is now settled. Both are right. Your genome is Nature and gives you a range of expressions open to you, and Nurture helps determine where along that continuum your expression lies. It's important to point out what a totally opposite view this is to what I learned in college genetics in the 1970s, because it's another example of how Science reverses itself without apology because it has based conclusions on incomplete evidence.

Epigenetics is of particular interest with respect to health. There are many factors that impact your gene expression. Beliefs and diet are two significant ones. But studies are showing—and scientists are surprised—that trauma not only affects genetic expression; those effects can be passed on for a number of generations. What this means to you in terms of health is that a trauma experienced by say, your great-grandmother, could be affecting your health and well-being today.

Most of the studies have been done on lab animals like mice and rats, but there are some studies on humans. It has been shown that descendants of Holocaust survivors have an 'abnormal' stress hormone profile, having less than normal amounts of cortisol, which is a hormone that helps with adaptation to stress.

Some studies show that epigenetic changes can be passed down through as many as 14 generations. The CDC, a bastion of establishment dogma, states that genetics account for only 10% of disease, with the remaining 90% owing to environmental variables. We are only beginning to understand the huge impact of environmental factors on health, but evidence indicates that they can affect not only you, but your offspring for generations.

Most of the time, you won't be aware of the trauma your ancestor experienced, or if you are, you might have no clue how it is affecting you, but don't worry. In the section on actions you can take, we will discuss some methods that might be useful for this problem.

The important point is that dis-ease is not solely caused by 'germs.' Your best protection from dis-ease is a strong energetic and physical body and a balanced mental-emotional condition. We can't avoid trauma, and we can't avoid ancestral effects, but there are ways to mitigate those effects. We'll talk about how in a later chapter.

~

Environmental Energy

There are some places on earth that are salubrious, while others are toxic. The most extreme are obvious even to an unconscious individual. Sacred spaces uplift and lighten your energy. Toxic waste dumps make you want to run screaming. There are many kinds of energies, and quite a few have a noxious effect on your health.

This book is not about space clearing. We have a *Busy Person's Guide* on that topic if you wish to investigate further; it's important you consider the energy at home and work when you are evaluating your health. Energy is invisible, but its effects can be devastating.

Symptoms of noxious energy run the gamut from simply annoying to life-threatening and can include just about anything from poor sleep to brain fog to cancer. The bottom line is that you need to be aware of environmental energies and cultivate healthy energy where you live and work.

We'll be mentioning some tips in the chapter on action items.

∼

Empathy & Boundaries

Empathy is knowing how another person is feeling, understanding their motives, being able to put yourself in their place. Most people regard empathy as a positive attribute, but often, it is detrimental, because highly empathic people tend not only to do the above, but also unwittingly take on other people's energies, and those energies can accumulate and lead to dis-ease.

The wounded healer is the most obvious example of a person being destroyed by empathy. But you don't have to be a professional healer to experience this syndrome. Many highly empathic persons were healers or shamans in past lives, and without even intending to, they take on noxious energies to help those they love. And because they are not trained in how to clear those energies, they often end up sick themselves.

We have seen dogs try to protect owners from noxious environmental energies by taking them on in much the same way, with very negative impact on their health.

Strong boundaries and empathy do not go hand in hand, and if you are highly empathic, you may find that you are sick more often than the average person and are depressed when you don't have a reason, because other people's energies become your own. I can remember being depressed one summer when I was a small child. Only many years later did I realize I was empathizing with my Mom, who was struggling with depression at that time. It felt like my depression, but it wasn't.

Learning to have appropriate boundaries and choosing not to take on other people's stuff can be very difficult for some people, but it is necessary if you want to live a healthy life.

~

The Subtle Energy Body

Your aura and chakras are vital parts of your subtle energy body, and if they are damaged, sooner or later your physical body will express that damage. All illness starts in the energetic body. By maintaining your aura and chakras, you head off physical dis-ease. And the good news is that it isn't that costly to learn basic techniques, as all of them depend on intention, and that doesn't cost you anything.

Your subtle body helps gather and direct energy into your physical body for vital life processes. When this connection is disturbed, ill health can develop. For chronically ill people, there are some patterns I have observed in myself and clients that could be considered a syndrome that keeps people trapped in ill health, no matter what they do. Since it relates to the energetic aspects of the body, we will discuss it here, even though it is not related to aura or chakras.

Early on in our business of helping clients—both animal and human —we discovered something thanks to a horse we were working on. When we muscle tested the horse, we got clear responses that pretty much indicated nothing at all was wrong with the animal. Yet it was obvious to both the owner and us that the horse was not doing well. Then we thought to dowse whether the horse's spirit was in its body, and the answer led us to a greater understanding of invisible factors that affect health.

Horses are prey animals, and as such, their response to fearful situations is to run away. If they cannot run away, or if they are feeling subjected to stress they cannot avoid, they do the next best thing. Their spirit leaves their body, 'spirit' meaning in this case the soul or incorporeal consciousness.

The spirit leaving the body is also seen in humans when they are subjected to abuse or serious stress. It can even happen if the person believes the world is a dangerous place or does not want to be here on earth in human form. It is surprisingly common in humans who have ill health for the spirit to be out of their body.

What we observed is that if the spirit is out of the body, nothing you do works to restore good health, so it is necessary to use intention to return the spirit to the body before you apply healing. Spirit being out of body also will give false answers to specific dowsing and muscle testing about health.

Dowsing is the best and easiest way to determine if the spirit is out of the body—you will get an accurate answer to this particular question, though you may be misled if you dive in and try to identify causes of health problems and solutions before checking on whether the spirit is out of body. See the Resources section for information on how to learn dowsing.

Intention usually puts the spirit back into the physical body, but if the major stress is still present, it will simply leave again, and we have observed that it can become a survival behavior in animals and humans, causing great resistance to healing efforts. Lowering stress and helping the person or animal to feel safe and think differently and eliminate stressors can help. So this is important to evaluate before investing lots of time and money into long-term health issues.

Grounding is an important aspect of having a healthy energy body, as is working to strengthen and balance all your major chakras and your aura. Good health begins in the energy body, so it pays to attend to it.

If grounding or keeping your spirit in your body is a challenge, try using crystal energy to help anchor your intention. There are many types of crystals that help with this. Pick one that has protective and grounding properties and is associated with the first chakra. I have found shungite works best for me, and there is a link in the Resources to my favorite source for shungite.

Your major chakras are associated with particular endocrine organs and their function, and if you have certain physical symptoms, it can point to a problem with a particular chakra. By working on that chakra, in addition to whatever else you do physically, you can speed recovery.

The aura is protective, and if it becomes damaged, your protection will be weakened. This can manifest in many ways, including lowered immunity. Aura damage can also present as physical symptoms, and when the damage is repaired, the physical symptoms often are resolved.

Tending to the health of your aura and chakras is a great first step to creating the health you desire.

∾

Stress

Stress in moderate amounts or acute stress, on rare occasions, are actually good things. That is probably because that is what the human body evolved to live with. Studies have shown that a certain amount of various types of stressors are actually helpful for the body, showing that humans not only adapted to natural stress, but harnessed it to make their bodies function better.

But the stress response and its benefits, as well as the definition of stress itself, are still undergoing study and change as scientists study the role of stress in health. One thing is becoming broadly accepted: that the constant stress of modern life leads to many negative health consequences. From heart disease in Type A individuals to digestive disorders that lead to obesity, cognitive function issues and other problems, stress creates a broad spectrum of ill health.

Ayurveda, a healing system developed 3000 years ago in India, believes that 85% of health problems start in the gut. The gut is amazingly vital for good health physically, mentally and emotionally. Stress causes good bacteria in your microbiome to die off and bad bacteria to multiply. Stress dries out your digestive tract, forcing the body to create more mucus in an attempt to rebalance, leading to permeability of the intestinal wall, then to all kinds of problems. Also, stress harms the function of your vagus nerve, causing many unpleasant symptoms. Finally, stress disrupts the balance of important hormones in your body, leading to poor sleep and digestive challenges. And these are merely a few of the known effects of stress.

If you live in an environment of high or constant stress, your health will pay the price. Your immune system goes haywire if it is overstressed or stressed unnaturally, but a certain amount of immune challenge helps you build immunity. What is the 'just right' point? The same answer we've been seeing all along. A natural amount in a natural way. And you are unique, so it isn't possible to say exactly. The good news is, you can learn to be aware of stress and then deal with it.

In a later chapter, we'll present some action items for helping you cope with stress in your life. For now, it is important to stop saying "It's all good" when it isn't. Don't paper over things that are causing you stress. Face up to them and then do something about them.

∼

Exercise

Take some time to examine your beliefs and attitudes. These are the most foundational aspects of good health and how hard or easy it will be for you to experience it. By changing what holds you back, you can see greater progress towards your health goals.

1. On a scale of 0-10, with 0 meaning you disagree completely and 10 that you agree completely, how much do you agree with the statement that good health requires a huge investment (time, money and/or effort)?
2. How much do you agree that your genes determine your health more than any other factor?
3. How much do you feel on a scale of 0-10 that you are a victim of what is going on outside of you? That you have no control over your health and are just a victim?
4. How strongly empathetic are you to what others feel and want from you?
5. How much effort or time or money do you put into maintaining or balancing your energy body (aura, chakras, energy in general) using any method?
6. How much stress do you have in your life? (Come on, be honest!)
7. How much negativity are you surrounded by or affected by from your family, friends and coworkers?
8. How hard does it feel to make changes in your health?

By consciously looking at the answers, you can see where you most need help or change.

6

TECHNOLOGY'S DANGERS

Introduction

One of the key aspects of modern living is the massive amount of technological change and scientific advances in the last hundred years. My Dad often talked about a fond memory he had as a boy of sitting on a hill above Boston harbor watching clipper ships sail in during the last days of sailing ships. People like my Dad, who was born in 1911, began life in a time when airplanes didn't exist and electrification of homes was uncommon in rural areas, and by the time they died, man had walked on the moon.

It is next to impossible for those of us who are younger to understand the huge progress that has been made technologically in our culture over the course of a single lifetime. We take it for granted. Yet historically speaking, this rapid pace of change is very unusual.

Believing that because a technological advance comes with benefits means it has no down side is a dangerous assumption. Living in a consumer society, we are constantly being bombarded with ads for the latest gadget or drug. The advertising emphasizes the benefits of the product and why you just have to have it. It doesn't even occur to us that maybe the product being sold to us isn't safe or doesn't work. We have become complacent, expecting the government to protect us from industrial greed or ignorance. Sadly, regulatory bodies and oversight committees are populated by special interests and bombarded by lobbyists to the point where if you don't watch out for yourself, you can have bad outcomes.

Those of us who grew up during the 60's remember ads for cigarettes showing doctors saying smoking had no negative health effects. Big Tobacco invested a great deal of money in suppressing the truth about cigarettes for many years, to the detriment of smokers. Big Pharma and the telecommunication companies are employing similar tactics in the present day to sell their products.

Technology offers us tremendous convenience and the ability to do things that are not 'normal' for humans. Planes fly us through the sky to whatever destination we choose; cell phones and the internet connect us with people far away; engineering marvels and modern sanitation allow humans to live in cities that have millions of people. These activities are not the natural human condition, and they offer a great deal of convenience, wonder and opportunity. But do they have a dark side?

In this chapter, we examine some of the negative outcomes of embracing technology without question or buying into the advertising for the latest gadget. While convenience is worth a price, maybe if that price is your health, you ought to reconsider the cost.

~

EMFs

Your body evolved to use natural electromagnetic fields (EMFs) to cue certain biological functions and to regulate certain processes. The sun and the cosmos are sources of natural EMFs to which your body responds and with which your body has evolved to interact in a positive fashion.

The proliferation of non-native EMFs in the 20th and 21st centuries appears to be a major contributing factor to what are called 'diseases of civilization,' that is, diseases that were not common in agricultural environments in the 19th century and earlier. It would be a mistake to blame every illness on EMFs, but we do feel strongly that if you eat and drink properly and attend to avoiding harmful EMFs, you will be addressing two of the biggest health problems modern man faces.

Manmade EMFs, also called non-native EMFs, present potential health problems for the very reason that your cells and your body have been tuned to respond to natural EMFs. It is hard for a young person today to comprehend the extent of electropollution, because what you grow up with, you take for granted as safe and normal. Our parents and grandparents lived in times when running water and electricity were not standard, yet by the time my Dad died, cell phones, computers, TVs and the electrification of residences was commonplace. This is an astounding amount of technological change. All of this technology produces EMFs that are not natural and that affect your body.

There are ample studies that demonstrate the negative effects of exposure to non-native EMFs. We suggest you research the database of curated articles at GreenMedInfo.com if you want to do a quick study. New research is coming in all the time to suggest that modern man is destroying his health with manmade EMFs. As we learn more about the electromagnetic aspects of the body and things like biophotons and the activity of mitochondria, it becomes possible to see how non-native EMFs are detrimental. There is little doubt that we have reached a point where most people are being exposed to too much radiation for too long.

The amount of profit at stake for the telecoms corporations is astonishing, and it leads to all kinds of questionable practices like disinformation campaigns and tobacco science-style research. Big

Pharma has exerted a great deal of pressure to get legislative protection in the US and to guarantee their profits; they certainly were more effective than Big Tobacco at reaching their goals. The telecoms companies are pressing towards their goals using methods that make Big Pharma look tame.

Many people are awakening to the health dangers posed by 5G systems, but are you aware that those closely spaced units on telephone poles that make 5G possible are not the last word in 5G? In 2018, the US FCC gave approval for a corporation to launch over 4000 satellites to begin to create a space-based network that will rain 5G radio frequencies down on everyone on earth. Ultimately, the plan is to have the planet covered with an array of 20,000 satellites constantly beaming 5G radiation everywhere on the planet. Not only does this project pose questions about space debris and atmospheric pollution, but it means there will be nowhere to hide from radiation that is designed to penetrate buildings and your body and has been shown to be harmful.

In the US, local and state governments have no right to opt out of 5G, so it will take massive reactions from the public to stop this type of electropollution. Neurologist Dr. Jack Kruse speculates that 5G will create such health problems that it will be impossible to ignore them for too long, but that won't help those who are affected. Dr. Joseph Mercola sees the EMF problem as a potential extinction event. Not since the Cold War and the fear of nuclear destruction has any single threat been so serious. Let's hope enough people awaken to this challenge and start taking action.

~

Visible Light Problems

Natural light is a specific type of electromagnetic radiation that your body has adapted to over eons. As with all natural phenomena, your body has developed ways to use natural light to enhance your health. Circadian rhythms are well known processes that depend on cues from natural, visible light, and they are found in many animals and plants.

The sun is our main source of visible light, and until fairly recently in history, the only other light sources man had were candles and fires, which were not very bright. But then gas lighting and electricity came along, and man was able to turn night into day.

There are convincing statistics to show that the electrification of houses correlated with increases in certain diseases. It is not known for sure why this is the case, but in addition to the concerns mentioned in the previous section, the alteration of light cycles probably had an effect. It is now thought that by reducing the production of melatonin, manmade lighting not only affects a person's ability to sleep well, but also impacts other rhythms and hormones which can lead to imbalances that explain the rise in diabetes and cancer, among other diseases.

Scientific studies make strong suggestions that two factors should be addressed: avoid blue light at the wrong time of day, and avoid manmade light for two to three hours before bedtime. Blue light is a particular frequency that is becoming a problem due to screens on computers, tablets, TVs and other devices. Your eyes are designed to react to the natural blue light that is common in the mornings. Blue light therefore is a trigger for helping you become active. It says 'daytime' to your body. And your body expects certain percentages of different color light at different times of day to cue different processes.

Computer screens and similar devices broadcast quite a bit of blue light, upsetting this natural balance. And the more we stare at screens at work and play, the more blue light we are exposed to. This messes up your circadian rhythms, and it has been shown to also lead to eye strain and may contribute to macular degeneration, in addition to leading to diabetes, obesity and other degenerative disorders. We will discuss measures you can take to protect yourself or mitigate these effects in the next chapter.

~

Drugs, Tests & Surgery

> One of the first duties of the physician is to educate the masses not to take medicine.
>
> -Sir William Osler

Drugs, tests and surgery are an integral part of modern medicine and a huge source of income for corporations, insurance companies and the government, directly and indirectly. While modern medicine excels in treating trauma, and sometimes in treating infection (though not always), it has an abominable record at treating other types of health problems. And in fact, it is becoming clear that modern medicine engages in practices that detract from overall health by harming the brain, the immune system and loading you with toxins, or creating side effects for which they then give you more drugs which don't solve the original problem.

> Whenever a doctor cannot do good, he must be kept from doing harm.
>
> -Hippocrates

As an aware person, you can choose how much and when to participate in this system. You can choose where to invest: in prevention or treatment. A natural approach would be to invest in good food and other things to boost your health and avoid needing professional care. This is not a pipe dream. Cultures other than our modern one achieve health and longevity in more natural ways. We recommend the video series *The Human Longevity Project*, listed in the resources, as a comprehensive look at the way a natural approach contributes to overall health and longevity.

When you do choose to take drugs, be empowered. The internet gives you the ability to look up drugs and their interactions and side effects. You will absolutely be amazed at how often a doctor will prescribe a drug that may not be a good idea for a patient. For example, when one tried to force chemotherapy on my Dad who did NOT have cancer, when he was in the hospital for pneumonia, and when the drug clearly states death is a side effect in the elderly. My Dad was 97 and had no cancer. Chemotherapy is a very lucrative type of drug to prescribe, and they did not inform us or my Dad before deciding to give it to him. We discovered the plan by accident. We complained to the hospital, but no action was taken against the doctor, an oncologist who was not my Dad's primary care physician, whom we had never even met. Why did he try to prescribe chemo? The only motivation we could find was it was billable on my Dad's great health insurance, and chemotherapy drugs at that time were a high ticket item in terms of profit. This is an example of a trend that is becoming worrying: the better your health insurance, the more the hospital is likely to do to you, whether you really need it or not. Informed consent is a thing of the past. Poor health insurance is presented as harmful to your health, but it turns out that isn't always so.

A good friend back in the 1980s lost her Dad because the family doctor switched him to a new heart med because of the convenience: it only had to be taken once a day, as opposed to his old prescription, which he had to take a few times daily. The doctor's motive was kindness, but he was misinformed and perhaps too busy to research for himself, instead listening to the drug rep's pitch. My friend's Dad was not the only person to die from taking that particular medicine. And it doesn't really matter how few die if your Dad is one of them.

Then there are drugs for less serious conditions than heart disease. Physical conditions like insomnia are not completely understood, so people resort to taking Ambien and other drugs to knock themselves out at night. The problem is that taking a drug shouldn't be a long term habit, and even taken short term, can have negative side effects, yet the number of people taking sleeping pills has grown alarmingly in recent years.

It isn't just physical conditions that are being handled in questionable ways with drugs. We know so little about how emotional and mental balance are created that it is egotistical to assume that current methods are perfect. We don't have a clear and complete picture about neurotransmitters and how they work, nor do we fully understand how the gut impacts your mental and emotional states, but we know that they do. In addition, the effect of diet and toxins is only beginning to be understood in terms of their role in causing dementia and autism.

Yet in spite of this ignorance, it has become commonplace to drug even children with psychoactive substances to suppress certain symptoms that are considered undesirable. Taking a pill seems so much easier than resolving the cause of 'bad' behavior, and it was a short step from prescribing Xanax, Ativan and Paxil for adults to doping children with what amounts to crystal meth. Sounds crazy, but at this time, children in the US are being prescribed Adderall, which is virtually the same drug as methamphetamine (an illegal drug sold as 'crystal meth'), with very similar actions and side effects. Even babies are being prescribed psychoactive drugs, and I can't get my head around how that can be justified.

Movies and books are an interesting source for observing trends in commonly accepted cultural behaviors. Look at movies from the 30s after Prohibition ended. The *Thin Man* series is an excellent example. The main characters are basically drinking alcohol constantly. To our current sensibilities, it is so extreme, it's laughable. Move on to the 40s and 50s, and your movie stars always seem to be smoking. You don't see tons of drinking and smoking in movies and books these days. Now you see characters mainlining

Diet Coke and taking anti-anxiety drugs and other prescription medications. These are the vices of our times, and like those of the past, such habits have a price in terms of health. Don't do what everyone else is doing without questioning how healthy it is. Just because it's legal and everyone is doing it doesn't mean you should, too.

It isn't just drugs you need to be concerned about. Medical tests can be invasive and dangerous. Don't submit to testing without making sure it is safe. The internet has lots of information. Sift through it with a critical eye. For example, some people die from reactions to dyes used in some imaging tests. Others have horrible results from tests like colonoscopy. Again, the number of deaths may be few, but if it's your Mom or grandchild that gets hurt or dies, it matters. Weigh carefully whether a test is worth the risk. Do your research online. A friend of ours had her heart damaged during a supposed 'routine' heart procedure, and it took an emotional as well as physical toll on her health, because the doctors admitted they couldn't fix the damage they had caused.

Surgery is always risky. My liver went south after my second 'routine' knee surgery because I reacted to the anesthesia they used. It took me years to get my health restored, and allopathic medicine was no help at all. Elective surgery should be considered carefully, and if you are a dowser, you should dowse about the outcome and side effects. It is possible to prepare yourself for surgery both physically and energetically to insure better results, but you won't be coached on that subject by an allopathic physician. You need to educate yourself. If I had been a dowser at that time, I would have known not to have the surgery, or what was needed to make it safe for me.

We tend to have a cavalier attitude about drugs, tests and surgery because they are so common, but they are not even remotely 'natural,' and they all have some degree of risk. When such things are the only way to restore your health or keep you healthy, fine, but don't approach tests, pills and surgery as if there is no risk. Be empowered. Research. Dowse. Choose what's best for you.

~

Vaccinations

Immunity depends on two systems: the innate and the adaptive systems. Innate immunity comes from elements always present and ready to fight, while adaptive immunity comes from a challenge to the system. Vaccinations are meant to stimulate activity on the part of the adaptive immune system.

Hypersensitivity and autoimmune disorders are rampant, and there are probably many contributing factors, but vaccination is probably one of them. The basic theory behind vaccination, that you stimulate an adaptive response to get the body to create antibodies to a particular disease, sounds totally rational. In practice, though, it isn't as easy to elicit a specific immune response as you might think. And that's probably all to the good. The hypersensitivity and autoimmune responses come from an immune system that has been stimulated too much or in the wrong way; we could even say, in an unnatural way.

Even the pharmaceutical companies admit vaccinations have side effects, and the side effects of vaccinations are easy to learn. Just read the insert that comes with the vaccine. Most are available online. The insert is the manufacturer's version of side effects, and you need to realize that if they are willing to be that honest about them, it isn't something to blow off. Bear in mind that the percent of cases of adverse reactions may appear very small compared to the actual incidence of adverse reactions due to the way studies are done.

Your adaptive immune system is designed to handle *natural* threats. In order to get it to respond artificially, vaccinations do something that is a huge no-no, and yet, it is rarely pointed out or talked about.

The huge no-no is that vaccinations inject things directly into your body, bypassing your body's natural processes and defenses.

Disease doesn't operate that way. To get sick, you breathe in or ingest something that leads to a response by your immune system. In many cases, the body will neutralize the threat, because the digestive tract is designed not to allow the wrong thing into your body. But if you inject something into the body, you are bypassing all the body's natural defenses, and the threat arrives in your bloodstream and cells as if out of nowhere. This is hardly a natural situation, and it certainly is not one your body was designed to respond to evolutionarily.

But even then, it is hard to get vaccines to work (defined as causing you to make antibodies) unless you use adjuvants; compounds to irritate and stimulate an immune response. Adjuvants like mercury in the form of thimerosal and aluminum and squalene are all known to be detrimental to health. Mercury and aluminum are known toxins that have adverse health effects, and toxins in general are particularly harmful to children. Children's immune systems are often less well-developed than adult immune systems; children's body size means they get greater exposure to toxins than adults; children are actively growing, and some types of toxic exposure do more damage to dividing cells.

Another issue is that some vaccinations use live viruses, which means you get injected with a live but supposedly less virulent form of a disease organism, and you will shed those live viruses for a period of time after you get your shot. In much the same way that parvo is spread among puppies, you spread shingles after your shingles shot. The polio shot has been shown to be the number one cause of polio cases, because it's risky using a live virus, because it's, well, alive.

Injecting people with toxins not surprisingly leads to brain damage (often called autism or autism spectrum disorder) and birth defects and immune issues like autoimmune disease, yet the vaccine manufacturers do their best to avoid admitting that. Billions have been paid in damages to US families with members killed or harmed irreparably by vaccinations, and that is the tip of the iceberg, because it is challenging to report vaccine issues and get reparations. For example, doctors apparently now say it's normal for babies to have seizures or cry for long periods of time after vaccination. Believe me, such behavior was nearly unheard of when I was a a child. Seizures and pain used to be considered a sign of a health challenge.

It has become crazy when obvious symptoms of ill health are termed 'normal' to defuse parents' concerns about the safety of vaccines. It reminds me of the time I spent at a vet's office volunteering, to see if I wanted to attend vet school. One morning, the vet was cropping puppies' tails. The puppies were very young, and he picked each one up and chopped off the tail with a scalpel, causing great wailing from the victims. When I asked him why he didn't use some kind of anesthetic, he said something like 'they don't feel pain,' or 'they're too young to have a well-developed pain response.' I asked him, "Then why are they howling when you do that?" He didn't have an answer and seemed offended that I had asked.

Similarly, if you are a mature woman, you might remember going in for a pelvic exam and being subjected to a freezing cold metal speculum and having the doctor reproach you for saying it felt awful, because he'd been taught you don't have feelings there. Even educated people like doctors can be programmed to believe the most illogical thing. You need to listen critically to what you are told by your doctor and vet, and you need to ask questions if it doesn't make sense.

On top of that, now doctors are 'incentivized' to make sure their patients are all vaccinated. A 2016 study showed that Blue Cross/Blue Shield, a major insurer, was incentivizing doctors to optimize children's vaccination schedules; if MDs met a target of 63% of eligible member patients, they received a payout of $400 per completed eligible member. This means your doctor is no longer an unbiased person to turn to for an opinion about vaccines. And it isn't the doctor's fault. Doctors are so busy trying to help their patients that they have little time for looking into conflicting theories about vaccinations, or to research side effects of drugs. They rely on the drug companies for information, and that information is hardly unbiased.

In order to convince yourself of the many dangers of vaccines, just download the insert from any common vaccine and read it carefully. While many downplay the percent of people who have adverse reactions, there are usually some scary potential adverse reactions, like death.

Furthermore, it clearly written on the inserts that vaccination does not guarantee effectiveness against the disease it is intended to prevent. Think what that means. You are accepting the potential for adverse reactions, including death in some cases, for the possibility, not the guarantee, of protection.

There is also the question of the optimal timing of vaccination administration. Since it is only logical that your immune system needs to be in good shape to respond to a vaccination and produce antibodies, you need to ask why patients in hospitals are being vaccinated, when they are sick or having major surgery or injured badly or recovering from general anesthesia. This is certainly a setup for creating weak or adverse reactions.

The only reason it is being done is that people in hospital rarely have their wits fully about them, and it is easier to say yes than to argue when you are lying in a hospital bed in a gown with no back to it, feeling miserable and powerless. I can remember even back in the 70s, veterinarians routinely vaccinated rescued animals before they had gained weight and become accustomed to their new homes. Frequently, these animals were (and still are) also subjected to flea dips and other pesticides when their bodies were in a very weakened condition.

The timing of insults to the body is a factor in the outcomes you see. A weakened, starved or sick body is not in any condition to respond well to toxic chemicals and immune system challenges. If doctors want vaccinations to work well, they should only be administered to people who are in relatively good health and not facing other health challenges.

Another issue is that a preponderance of vaccine studies have bad experimental models, and thus yield faulty conclusions. Even in high school, you learned that a control group is different from a test group in that the control group doesn't get anything that changes or threatens to change the status quo. Sugar pills and salt water shots are an example of control group treatments.

In modern vaccine studies, the test subjects get the new shot, while the 'control' group gets a different shot, one that is deemed 'safe.' Sometimes, the control group just gets the 'inactive' ingredients of the same shot, or those deemed inactive. How is that good science? It isn't. Those supposedly inactive ingredients include contaminants and adjuvants. This type of bad science does indeed cause misleading results that appear to support the efficacy or safety of vaccines in some cases, which is of course why the studies are being done this way.

Long terms studies? Studies on receiving multiple shots in quick succession? They aren't done. Yet in recent decades, the number of shots for children has increased dramatically, along with increases in autism, allergies and autoimmune disorders. Shouldn't someone be interested?

You are interested. If you have children or pets, they are going to be subject to untested and dangerous vaccine policies that are driven by profit. The number of recommended vaccines for children went up dramatically after vaccine makers got a law passed to give them immunity from prosecution in the US. This is not a coincidence.

The key point of giving vaccinations is to trick the body into producing antibodies, because current science says that antibodies means you have immunity. However, there are many scientists who question this assumption, saying that having antibodies only proves you were exposed to a disease previously; it is not a measure or guarantee that you could fight off that disease if exposed in the future. This is a huge gap in the rational explanation of how vaccinations work. All vaccinations are designed to do is make you produce antibodies, but that isn't the same as making you truly immune to disease.

Herd immunity is totally unproven, as recent outbreaks of disease in fully vaccinated populations prove, yet often, that weak argument is trotted out as a way to create fear and judgment towards unvaccinated individuals. Vaccines, in spite of the hype, are not 100%. If pressed, your doctor or vet will admit that.

Living in crowded environments is a major risk factor for disease. Before sanitation was good, water sources were often polluted, and poor city dwellers with malnourished bodies fell prey to diseases of all kinds. Modern sanitation has improved living conditions and safety. This has been a key factor in the reduction of epidemics like smallpox, but medical science likes to claim vaccination is the cause.

Another factor not often discussed is that when a new disease hits the scene, it is often virulent, but over time, probably since microorganisms evolve so quickly, it becomes less virulent and morbidity and mortality tend to decline, because it really isn't in the best interest of a disease organism to kill its host. In fact, both disease organism and host evolve over time to create a more harmonious balance. An example is that having chicken pox as a child appears to protect you from shingles as an adult. Shingles has become rampant in part because of the suppression of chicken pox, but also because the shingles vaccine is usually a live virus, and the virus sheds for a time after vaccination, creating the potential for infecting other people. Diseases that are not life-threatening, like measles and chicken pox, stimulate a proper immune response and often confer a health benefit. It is therefore questionable science to subject anyone to vaccination for a nonlethal disease.

Similarly to having chicken pox conferring some immunity to another disease, in this case, shingles, it appears that a vaccination can have as an unwanted side effect the stimulation of another disease in the vaccinated person. Historically, it has been postulated that the smallpox vaccine led to cases of tuberculosis and syphilis in the vaccinated. Some scientists theorize that the rise in cancer in modern society may be related to the increase in vaccinations. Whether these cases are a side effect caused by contaminants in the vaccine or by a miscued immune system is not yet known. More studies need to be done, but it's unlikely pharmaceutical companies will fund them.

The US Supreme Court has ruled vaccines to be "unavoidably unsafe." When you combine that with over $4 billion in vaccine injury payments as of 2018, it is pretty obvious that vaccines are not as safe as the manufacturers want you to believe.

There is a lot of propaganda, social pressure and bad science out there about vaccines, but there are also many scientific studies and books that expose the truth.

Vaccination has become a procedure that in the US, you are authorizing when you sign a hospital admittance form. The form won't say vaccinations; it uses a euphemism. For many years now, hospitals have been administering vaccinations to patients when they are in the hospital for unrelated procedures and illnesses. Logic would point out that the absolute wrong time to get a vaccine is when your system is stressed from recent surgery, your liver is detoxing general anesthesia, or you are ill with another ailment, yet that doesn't seem to stop this practice.

My father in the 1980s went into the hospital for a 'routine' prostate surgery which required general anesthetic. While he was there, they talked him into getting a pneumonia shot. Shortly thereafter, he developed cold antibody disease, a hemolytic anemia. His red blood cells would clot and burst when he became cold. The doctors called it 'idiopathic,' meaning they didn't have a clue what caused it. Autoimmune issues often do show up after vaccination. The interesting fact is that my Dad had to move to a warmer climate because of this condition, a very stressful and unhappy choice for him and my Mom, and when he went into the hospital the last time before he died, nearly 25 years later, he went in with....pneumonia.

There is plenty of real information available on vaccinations, but you cannot get your facts from mainstream media, sellers of vaccines like the CDC and drug companies, or even state and federal governments. You need to educate yourself and make informed decisions. The rise in terrible side effects, most of all, brain damage and autoimmune disease, are leading to a major health crisis in the future in this country, because the health care system cannot survive if there aren't enough people working and paying taxes to support it.

A good health care system should make more people well, not chronically ill. Studies routinely show that the US, with the highest vaccination rates in the world, has higher autism rates than other developed countries and much higher under age 5 mortality rates. This was not true before vaccinations became so prevalent. Yet in spite of these data, there is much media and legislative pressure to increase the number of mandatory vaccinations children get in the US.

~

Negative Nutrition

We've addressed the critical nature of eating good food if you want to be healthy. There is no single physical thing more important to your health than eating and assimilating nutritious food. There are many cultural challenges to this vital function. Fast food, junk food and stress lead to very poor eating habits. The perception that you don't have time causes you to rush through or skip meals, contributing to the problem. You are attracted to foods that resonate with your energy, and if you are loaded with negative energies, it is very hard to force yourself to eat 'right.' Stress makes it hard to digest your food adequately. Our culture has moved away from making meal time a time of love and gratitude and positive social interactions, which erodes the process further.

Technology adds to this burden. Pesticides cause all kinds of damage to your gut microbiota, as well as disrupting important biological processes and being toxic to your system.

GMOs are even more troubling. As Dr. John Douillard, an expert on Ayurveda, points out in an article on his lifespa.com website:

> New research has found that bacteria in our guts are like Velcro for picking up new genetic material, which is then passed on to the human genome, which could then potentially affect how our genes express themselves. Many researchers now believe that this process of horizontal gene transfer is one of the main drivers for human adaptation and/or evolution. **Moreover, there is much concern now about how altered DNA from genetically modified (GMO) foods is impacting the human genome and its expression.**

Recent studies therefore suggest that there could be gene transfer between humans and GMO foods, leading to unknown consequences.

Another unfortunate technological development driven by greed is the use of toxic biosludge as 'fertilizer' on crops you eat. The EPA in the US has approved the spraying of toxic biosludge on food crops as fertilizer, in spite of the fact that it is loaded with heavy metals and pharmaceutical drug residues. Just as we would not suggest the use of animal manure on your garden if those animals have been fed GMO feeds or treated with antibiotics, hormones and pesticides, we are horrified that the EPA would consider biosludge a legitimate fertilizer. It reminds me of when ketchup was classified by the government years ago as a vegetable for the purposes of pretending school lunches were healthy.

Just as dangerous and scary, but not getting as much notice in the media, is the destruction of soils. Agribusiness doesn't tend to soil health at all, and yet it's the soil organisms that help make your food healthy. Microorganisms like bacteria and fungi are required for healthy soil, but even one application of Roundup can seriously alter the soil microbiota, much as a round of antibiotics can disturb the healthy function of your gut. So it isn't only that soils are being depleted of minerals because of current farming practices; the soil organisms are destroyed with glyphosate (the key ingredient in Roundup, which is used extensively on GMO crops) and other pesticides, and it's those organisms that are largely responsible for making our food healthy and compatible with human digestion. Glyphosate has contaminated the ground water and even the air in some locations, and it is vital that its use be outlawed if we want to have any hope of producing decent food in the future.

~

Geoengineering & Aerosol Spraying

The subject of air pollution was a hot topic when I was growing up, and there have been many laws passed to attempt to improve the quality of the air we breathe. That's why it's strange that the phenomenon of geoengineering is proceeding at such an intense pace with so few people even being aware of it.

Geoengineering is not a new science. Even fifty years ago, there was research being done on how to create certain types of weather conditions artificially. The space race and the rise of technology put this subject into the lap of the military. From star wars defense systems to controlling the weather in battle conditions, 'black' projects concerning geoengineering and atmospheric modification appear to have proliferated in this century.

Your tax dollars are being used in this type of work, which has clearly proceeded beyond the lab. Jets are spraying materials of uncertain chemical composition in the skies, as evidenced by the lingering white lines in checkerboard patterns that blend into an unnatural type of overcast within 24 hours after spraying. You Tube has plenty of videos showing that this is taking place worldwide, and yet it is hard to guess what the purpose is. It must cost a ton of money, and it's being denied and done in secret, so it makes sense that it must have a military application. At the very least, it isn't for your good, or they'd be rushing to claim credit.

An incredible amount of effort is being put into denial and discrediting those who talk about this subject, but as an aware individual who cares about health, it behooves you to be aware that this is going on not only in the US, but in other countries as well, and that there is absolutely no science at all on the health effects of this practice. Other than joining the ranks of believers, there isn't much at this point you can do about this phenomenon, but if you have breathing issues, you may want to curtail your outside activity on days when aerosol spraying is being done.

~

Water Pollution

Many people live in areas that depend on city water sources. Others have wells or in rare cases, springs from which to draw water. While even natural sources of water can have contaminants like arsenic or pesticides from nearby agricultural runoff, city water or tap water is far more likely to be unhealthy and unnatural.

Tap water has chlorine in it, because they want to kill germs. Remember the Germ Theory of Disease? That all germs are bad for you? But it's wrong? Obviously, you don't want to drink water full of microorganisms, but if you chlorinate water to kill them and then drink or bathe in the chlorinated water, how does that affect your gut and skin microbiota? Not in a good way, that's for sure.

An example of how it is natural to use one's senses came in the case of my sister's dog. My sister lived in a suburb of Salt Lake City, Utah on city water. The water was so awful that she bought bottled water for the family. One day when I was visiting, she commented that her dog drank very little water, and since they lived in the desert, she thought this was odd. (A female dog they had prior to the male dog had a horrible bladder stone, which may or may not have been from drinking or not drinking tap water.) When she confessed that only the humans got bottled water, I replaced the dog's water with bottled water and put the dish on the floor. He immediately drank a whole bowl. The nose knows, as they say, and dogs are loath to drink 'bad' water. But dehydration, as we pointed out earlier, leads to disease symptoms of all kinds. So make sure your pets get good water, too.

It is important to be aware of the quality of the water you drink, cook with and bathe in. Filters of all kinds abound, and it is worthwhile to investigate the best filter for your needs. You can get filters for your shower head and your kitchen tap. You can use a pitcher filter. Or you can get a filtration system to put under your sink.

Bottom line is that in most areas, tap water in not healthy to drink. I can remember visiting my parents in the Phoenix area years ago. They were living in Tolleson, which was then located near a lot of agricultural fields that produced cotton, citrus and roses. The water that came out of their tap was cloudy and smelled and tasted awful. I am not making this up! I am sure it had runoff of pesticides and all kinds of stuff.

Nowadays, they are finding drugs and drug metabolites in city water. My mother was told to flush her fentanyl patch after use. That's right. Flush the opioid drug down the toilet. Where do you suppose that drug ended up? And drug metabolites (breakdown products) from users? Where do they end up? This is not a trivial concern.

So it is vital that you be alert to the quality of your water and take whatever measures you need to assure it is pure and safe.

~

Information Overload

In Nature several thousand years ago, which isn't that long in terms of evolutionary or geologic time, most humans lived in small, family-oriented communities and had only moderate or rare communication outside of their 'tribe.' Even in the early 20th Century, there were many in the US and other 'first world' countries who didn't have frequent communication outside of their immediate area.

Then came telephones, telegraph, television, the internet, radio, email and suddenly, the world was connected. It is hard for us to picture how different life would be if we didn't have radio, TV, the internet, email and telephones. One thing is for certain. These technologies are now flooding you with information.

You get notification of events around the world, most of them negative. "If it bleeds, it leads." And you are bombarded with advertising that tells you that you absolutely must buy this or that to be healthy, wealthy and happy. It is not natural to have negative information and advertising constantly pouring into you. It leads to overwhelm and stress.

Technology has brought a lot of convenience, but the amount of information in modern life is way more than you were designed to be exposed to. Phone calls are cheap and easy. You can stay in touch with loved ones, whereas in the past, an infrequent letter was all you could count on. But there are many down sides to this level of connection and to the negative slant with which most news and information is presented. Fear is a great motivator, and it is used blatantly in the news and even in advertising. Fear leads to stress, and stress causes ill health.

Some people are now choosing to disconnect from this constant bombardment. They realize the news is so filtered and negative, it isn't really beneficial. They are tired of constant spamming emails, nastiness on social media and above all, the massive amount of selling they are forced to submit to.

How connected you are is a choice. While connection brings some convenience, you must weigh how much connection you really need. When I was a kid, we didn't own cell phones, and yet we were just fine. Most of these conveniences are only truly useful in emergency situations, and those are rare. Don't assume just because everyone is doing something or everyone has something means you must, too.

~

Exercise

On a scale of 0-10, how strongly do you feel the following are impacting your health in a negative way:

1. Putting convenience, money and expediency as priorities. Making excuses for not changing.
2. EMFs and blue light issues at home and work.
3. Using prescription or other drugs; getting any vaccination the doctor suggests for you, your children, your pets
4. Eating foods that are lacking in nutrition and vitality or contain toxins, or both; drinking liquids that are harmful or not helpful to good health
5. Spending too much time sitting; not getting enough exercise
6. Lacking exposure to fresh air and sunlight

For those that you assigned a number of 8 or higher, it would be good to start taking action to reduce the impact by looking at the chapter on action steps.

Don't be discouraged by the vast number of ways that technology can harm your health. There are ways that a conscious person can improve their physical health, in spite of the fact that we are bombarded by our culture with so many potentially harmful choices about food, behavior and the environment.

You have the ability to create the health you want, but it will perhaps require a greater level of consciousness than you are comfortable with, and it will certainly involve shifting your outlook to a more empowered one.

In the next chapter, we discuss a starting point for empowered natural health, and after that, we look at the many positive actions you can take to improve your chances of reaching your health goals.

7

TAKING ACTION

Introduction

This is the chapter where we make concrete suggestions that we
believe will improve your health and that are in alignment with the
values of natural health. The thing about natural health is that it is,
well, natural, which means anyone can do it. Sure, you may need to
consult a health care professional now and then, but it is only in
modern times that people have been led to believe that health is
completely in the hands of their doctors instead of themselves. By
applying natural health principles, you can head off a lot of health
challenges and even resolve some on your own with a lot less
financial cost than consulting professionals.

It goes without saying that if you have a longstanding or serious
health condition, you should always get professional help, but if you
are in overall good health, you can apply natural health methods and
expect to see improvement, and often, that improvement won't be
exactly what you expected, because everything is interconnected,
and healing often brings surprising or totally unexpected positive
outcomes.

There are so many free and inexpensive ways you can improve your health by changing your thoughts, detoxing occasionally, getting good sleep, breathing properly, moving your body in natural ways and restoring your gut microbiome by eating well. A great deal of improvement can be seen by eliminating certain habits, which can also end up saving you money in the long run.

The beauty of applying natural suggestions is that in many cases, they involve not money, but merely time and effort. Remember, you cannot expect change without changing, and this chapter will give you actionable tips that almost anyone can apply with minimal investment, except maybe if you are eating a really bad diet and decide to upgrade that. Good food isn't cheap. But even for that, the money you save by eliminating unhealthful practices could balance that investment.

Be aware that you won't be able to completely recreate a natural existence. As Bill Bryson points out in his book *At Home,* life for humans changed radically 10,000-15,000 years ago when we turned from being hunter-gatherers to living a more sedentary lifestyle, relying on agriculture and living in crowded conditions. He says:

> A typical hunter-gatherer enjoyed a more varied diet and consumed more protein and calories than settled people, and took in five times as much vitamin C as the average person today. Even in the bitterest depths of the ice ages, we now know, nomadic people ate surprisingly well—and surprisingly healthily. Settled people, by contrast, became reliant on a much smaller range of foods, which all but ensured dietary insufficiencies...So sedentism meant poorer diets, more illness, lots of toothache and gum disease, and earlier deaths. What is truly extraordinary is that these are all still factors in our lives today.

Very few people can or will choose to revert to a Paleolithic lifestyle. We're not saying you should. However, being aware of the challenges of the way we live as modern humans allows us to take action to mitigate negative effects and improve our health. In this chapter, we discuss mainly simple steps, many of which don't cost much, that will align you with a more natural and healthy way of living.

The basic thrust of this approach is to examine what you are doing, how you are living and how you think and ask yourself, "Is this natural?" Then ask yourself, "How can I live a more natural life and still get the outcomes I want?"

The word 'natural' is overused and misused in advertising, because people in most cases desire a more natural experience, so you see "Nature" and "Natural" in many brand names of foods and supplements. Unfortunately, there are no hard and fast legal definitions of the words, and that means advertisers can use them however they see fit. And it isn't all their fault, because when you think about it, what is 'natural'? You can call water from a mountain stream natural, but if a mining operation upstream has polluted it with heavy metals, is it still in a natural condition, even though it is in Nature? What about chemicals in personal care products, where the seller goes to great lengths to show the ingredients are natural by saying this chemical is derived from coconuts, and that one is derived from flowers? How much processing can a natural substance undergo before it is no longer natural?

The point is that you absolutely cannot trust advertising to make your choices. For your health, the closer to the form found in Nature, unspoiled and unprocessed, the more natural something is. The closer you can get to that kind of natural, the healthier in most cases. So organic coconut oil is more natural than a chemical you cannot pronounce that is derived from coconuts. Unprocessed is always more natural than processed. A vitamin or mineral you get from food is always more natural than taking a pill. Sunlight taken outdoors is more natural than a light from a tanning bed or full spectrum lightbulbs. Manmade technological substitutes like electric lights and gadgets are not natural.

Modern humans are far removed from a natural lifestyle at this point, so no matter what you do, you won't have a fully natural lifestyle, but by making the most natural choices you can, you improve your chances of creating good health. So, as you make those choices, you ask 'is this natural?' rather than accepting advertising or someone's word for it. You do your own thinking and research to verify your choice.

There are three general types of situations that occur when you ask and answer those questions. The first type is when you find you can tweak what you are doing, as in eating a better diet or learning to meditate or going to bed earlier. Those situations—and there will be many of them—are simply a matter of you altering your lifestyle a little bit, of investing a little time and effort or a bit of money.

But other times, you will find yourself perhaps challenged to find a way to live more naturally and still get your desired outcome. These situations are more challenging, because they are the times you may have to give up some things you are addicted to, or which you may think you cannot live without. Examples of that are your smartphone and the habit of staring at all kinds of screens like your computer, TV and tablet or using electric lights at night. Only you can decide if the benefits are worth the cost. We think they are, but it's your choice.

The third type of situation is when you find something that is not subject to your control, or that you could theoretically control, but don't have the resources to do so. An example of this would be if you discover your house has a bad case of dirty electricity or you are living next door to a cell tower or your workspace is awash with noxious EMFs. The cost to repair the electrical issues or move or get a new job is a huge investment indeed, and not one to take lightly. Yet, by becoming aware that those things could be contributing significantly to eroding your health, you at least have a choice to address the situation or not. We do not believe that ignorance is blissful. Living in ignorance has only bad outcomes, so being aware is a blessing. We believe in the support of the Universe in these situations, and we urge you to ask for help and expect it.

We suggest that you start with simple things that you can easily change and work up to the bigger ones, because success will breed confidence and help you to make the next decision and the next one. Don't try to do it all at once, and don't tackle something too scary or too big, because that is a type of self-sabotage.

We present a variety of useful things you can do in this chapter, but we do not include training. We trust you can get online and do research about any technique or suggestion that resonates with you. Usually, there are books, free articles and other economical resources.

∾

Your Approach To Natural Health

You've read about a wealth of challenges to health that are part of everyday living, many of them manmade and of recent origin. Yet so many of these things are now accepted as 'natural,' as part of life. How can you hope to overcome those issues without putting yourself back in the Stone Age?

There has been so much progress in the last hundred or so years that it is unthinkable to walk away from it. You don't want to go back to splitting wood to heat your home, to using an outhouse or growing all your own food, any more than you want to throw away your phone or car.

While it is true that eliminating all sources of health problems would put you back into a lifestyle common 150 years ago, the past had its own challenges, and if you react in fear, without thought, you would just be swapping one set of problems for another. As humans, we are always looking for the quick fix and for someone to tell us what to do, and that leads to problems, no matter what time you live in.

Going back in time isn't the answer to the challenges of natural health; using critical thinking and your intuition are.

Empowered natural health means becoming aware of the many choices you are faced with and making what you feel are the best ones for you. You can mitigate harmful effects without totally turning away from modern convenience. In order to succeed, it will be helpful if you adopt certain beliefs and attitudes.

~

Avoidance And Fear

We talked about obvious toxins in the environment and that you should avoid them. But is avoidance always a solution? It depends. Avoiding toxins like non-native EMFs and toxic metals like mercury and aluminum, and pollutants like pesticides is a good idea. But avoidance is just one useful strategy, and it should be employed mainly with regard to things which are uniformly harmful to humans.

But too often, people tend to use avoidance as a broad strategy, and it ends up making them live in fear and feel like even natural elements of their environment are their enemies. Avoiding one type of food forever does not heal problems like food allergies, for example. It just eliminates the symptoms, but the symptoms were signs of an underlying imbalance or insufficiency. Address that deficiency, and in many cases, the food item can be eaten at some point with impunity. In other words, sometimes avoidance is a good temporary strategy, but you need to address underlying issues to allow your body to become whole.

So while natural health would demand that we avoid unnatural things like GMOs, avoidance should be combined with positive action that you believe will help you reach your goals. If you find yourself living in fear and focusing on what you are afraid of, it's time to shift your focus to things you can control that are helpful for your health goals.

~

No Silver Bullets

Creating optimal health and longevity is a journey. You can't take a pill. You can't even just follow a certain diet and expect total success. Health involves all the factors we've discussed, which means you need to become conscious of how you are thinking, feeling, acting, etc. You have to look at all aspects of life, from thoughts to actions to eating plans and exercise and what's in your environment. Even if you do that, you must remember how little we know about how the human body works. When working with only a small portion of the complete knowledge required to create good health, following a natural model makes a lot of rational sense.

Take your time. The journey will teach you so much. And every step of the way, you can improve your health. Put aside impatience and laziness. Be willing to commit time, effort and even money as needed. There are no magic pills or silver bullets that will give you good health, but your goals are attainable.

~

You Are Unique

You know that you are unique. Sure, you are human, and many general things that affect all humans will apply to you. But since health is intimately tied to how you think and believe, and it is strongly related to your energies, your health journey will be unique.

There is no one-size-fits-all strategy for good health. Even applying the idea of living a more natural life will need to be tweaked to suit your energies, your beliefs, your lifestyle. It becomes a journey of self-awareness and discovery as you build good health. And it can even be enjoyable.

Don't become discouraged that what works for others doesn't work for you. We have all faced this challenge. It is not a sign that you are defective, nor is it a sign that you are inadequate to the task. If you are determined to create a naturally healthy lifestyle, and you don't give up, you will eventually succeed. Be flexible. Be optimistic.

∼

Don't Be Overwhelmed

Natural health is simply living as naturally as possible, as close to what Nature intended as you are able to. It may seem overwhelming to have to examine all aspects of your life, from your job to your living space to how you eat, and so on, because you are looking at your whole life.

Don't allow yourself to become paralyzed by the sheer scope of the challenge. Just start at an obvious point for you, and keep expanding into other areas of life until you feel you have done what you can. Don't get fearful or negative, because you have access to all the tools and information you need to make changes that will help you live a more natural, healthy life.

∼

Food

Eating good quality food is vital to your health, but if you have digestive issues, just switching to a better diet may not fix them. If you have leaky gut or food allergies or an unbalanced or deficient gut microbiota, you may need to resolve conditions like inflammation and repopulate your gut microbiota before you will see significant progress.

If you have any major digestive issues, consult a holistic doctor, because you are unique and there are no one-size-fits-all solutions. But in general, she will probably tell you to eliminate toxins and allergens from your diet and do something to heal the gut.

Deglycyrrhizinated licorice, or DGL, was very useful to me in my healing process. Another herbal option is to go with a slippery elm/marshmallow/licorice preparation like you can find at Dr. John Douillard's store online. Basically, you need to soothe the gut lining and allow it to repair, and there are many options for that purpose.

Creating conditions which will encourage good health include making sure you have microorganisms in the right number and with the right amount of diversity to digest your food and assimilate it. Your doctor will make suggestions about the best probiotic for repopulating your gut, or you can dowse or select one of the better brands available at the whole foods store. We'll talk more about microbiomes in the next section.

Choosing the right diet depends on your needs, but we found the ancestral/paleo diet was good for resetting our hormones and helping us drop cravings and snacking. Eliminating grains and going organic and unprocessed is a good way to take stress off your digestion, as it mimics a paleolithic diet. We now eat a modified Paleo diet that includes a small amount of organic oatmeal and organic Einkorn flour. Einkorn is the oldest wheat, and due to its unique properties, many people who can't tolerate wheat or think they are gluten sensitive eat Einkorn just fine, like I do.

The fact that gluten intolerance is rampant in the US and that gluten intolerant people can eat wheat products in Europe in many cases indicates this problem is not simply one of gluten, since all wheat has gluten. Probably, the issue is more complex and may in part be confused due to focusing on gluten, which isn't really a single definable substance that is always the same. Gluten is a substance that varies from wheat to wheat and grain to grain, and that makes it very hard to pin down gluten's health effects and verify them.

Most grain flours have gluten, which is a mixture of various proteins formed when water is mixed with the flour. The key is this: gluten is not a single type of molecule or substance, and it varies from one type of wheat to another. Einkorn flour actually has more protein than most grains, but the gluten formed by einkorn flour contains more low molecular weight proteins than other wheat flours, and if you try to cook with it, you will easily recognize the difference this makes, because it is a little more challenging to use in baking. So the ability of some people to tolerate einkorn flour is probably not because it has less gluten; it's because the gluten has a different composition.

There are those who pooh-pooh the gluten-free movement as a fad and make fun of those who avoid grains because of gluten. This is because there is still a lot to learn about the effects of grains on our metabolism and health and because of that, reactions are not uniform or predictable from person to person. For example, some people who have terrible reactions to wheat in the US often find that they can tolerate wheat products when traveling in the UK. This would seem to add fuel to the skeptics' point of view, but that's only because you can't uniformly condemn all gluten and predict a reaction, because glutens vary so much.

Certainly, it has been shown that it is wise to significantly reduce the amount of grains in your diet and to make sure those you ingest are organic, gluten or not. Unless you have been diagnosed with celiac sprue, you can experiment with grains to find if you are intolerant to gluten, or simply intolerant to the highly hybridized forms of wheat being used today, the pesticides used to raise wheat, or the high molecular weight proteins in the gluten of different types of wheat. Some people will see drastic improvement simply by going organic, because pesticides can be a major culprit for some people who have food reactions. Next, try flours like Einkorn and various heirloom varieties which have not been hybridized or genetically modified. We have some links in the Resources for you to explore. Be aware that products marked 'gluten-free' are processed and not necessarily organic and might even contain GMOs, so mindlessly going to a gluten-free diet is not really the way to go in any case. If you choose to eliminate all gluten, make sure you limit grains and grain products in your diet and only use organic for best results.

Fermented foods, if you are not histamine sensitive, are a gold mine for creating good digestion. Each type of fermented food has its own microbiota, and you can help the diversity in your gut by sampling many, from kefir drinks to yogurt to sauerkraut. Making your own fermented foods from local ingredients is even better, as it gives your gut the right local microbes for good health. Your gut microbiome thrives if it has the right amount of the right types of gut microorganisms, and fermented foods are a great source.

Eat organic, non-GMO food. If 99% of your body's functions are coded by bacterial and viral DNA, how wise is it to eat fake foods made using bits of viral and bacterial DNA that then end up inside your body? Natural is best.

Even the best diet will require some supplementation, so use your judgment and add supplements according to the earlier chapter on that topic. Get high quality, bioavailable products with minimal additives and binders.

If possible, get your nutrients from real food. For example, real salt has trace minerals not found in grocery store iodized salt. The different colors of Himalayan, Celtic and Redmond salt are signs of their different mineral compositions. Natural salt is vital for health, and it doesn't have the negative health effects of 'fake' salt. A salt-free diet is actually not healthy. Real salt provides many health benefits, and in fact is so valuable that it was once used to pay Roman soldiers. Thus the word 'salary,' which comes from the Latin word for salt. You couldn't pay anyone in grocery store salt, and now that natural salt is readily available, it can't be used as money, but it still holds great health value. Switch to a real salt product and use it regularly. If you have doubts, read Dr. David Brownstein's book *Salt Your Way To Health* and learn how critical it is for your health.

Iodine is another mineral we all need. A deficiency of this substance is implicated in many conditions. We use an organic kelp seasoning to make sure we get our iodine. It's easy to use along with salt. Preferably get a product that is organic and doesn't come from the Pacific ocean (we have concerns about the effects of Fukushima's radiation on products from the Pacific). There is a link to the product we use in the Resources section, along with a link to Dr. David Brownstein's website. His book on iodine is an eye-opener. Getting enough iodine in your diet also provides a measure of protection against various radiation exposures. A side note: the breads you buy in the store often contain brominated flour, meaning the flours contain the element bromine, which is used to enhance the action of gluten. Bromine attaches to receptors in the thyroid for iodine, suppressing proper function. Bromine is a known endocrine disruptor. It is also potentially a carcinogen. Limit grain intake; bake your own bread or at least research brands and avoid brominated flours.

A special note on artificial sweeteners is in order. I can't believe ANYONE is drinking diet sodas and using aspartame. In the 1980s, while I worked at NASA, we read an article in the local paper saying studies showed bad health effects from drinking diet sodas. We all quit. More studies have been done since then, yet somehow, the word doesn't doesn't seem to have gotten out.

Artificial sweeteners are bad for you in large part because they taste sweet, but aren't sugar. Your body tastes sweet and assumes sugar is coming. Natural sugar. It gears up to metabolize sugar, and then it gets....none. Weight gain is a proven side effect of artificial sweetener consumption. Insulin resistance develops, adding to the diabetes epidemic.

Raw honey is fine as a sweetener in moderation. Anything processed is not as good for you, and the more processed and less natural, the worse it is. High fructose corn syrup is terrible. Aspartame should be outlawed. Minimize your intake of sugar and just don't use substitutes.

Another problem is the use of microwaves. Microwaving food is not a good idea, as it can create carcinogenic substances. Heat or cook your food in a toaster oven or regular oven, not the microwave. Get rid of the microwave altogether, as it puts out non-native EMFs.

Drink more pure water and less of other beverages. The chlorine in tap water is not good for your gut microbiota, so filter tap water if you must use it for drinking and cooking. Consume caffeine and alcohol in moderation, and even less if you have vagus nerve issues, as they can irritate the vagus nerve.

Removing foods from your diet may be necessary as a stopgap measure, but aim to heal your gut and be able to eat just about anything at some future point. Eating fewer and fewer foods actually is bad for your gut microbiota. A variety of good foods is beneficial.

Try to have a ritual such as a blessing before you eat and make your meal a happy time. Enjoy eating, and you are helping balance your lower chakras. Practicing gratitude is also healing. If you find yourself rushing to eat and not chewing and not enjoying it, you may have some beliefs you need to shift.

A certain amount of fasting is beneficial. Try to eat your largest meal at midday and don't eat within three hours of bedtime. If you can leave a long period between your last meal one day and your first the next, you have given your system time to heal and repair. If you snack in the evenings, your body has to digest instead.

This covers some actions you can take to improve your health by eating and drinking more naturally. In the next section, we will discuss things you can do to support your microbiota.

Microbiota: Skin

Your skin, even places like your eyeballs, have their own array of microorganisms who live in harmony with your skin cells, performing many valuable functions. When you take a shower with chlorinated tap water or swim in a pool, use sunscreen, dye your hair or use antibiotic wipes, you are harming your skin's friendly microorganisms.

Support your skin microbiota by using only natural products for personal care. Deodorant, shampoo, skin lotion: these products now mostly contain a ton of chemicals. Even those claiming to be natural are not.

Use coconut oil instead of sunscreens and avoid excessive exposure to the sun. The SPF of almond or coconut oil is good enough if you don't stay out too long. And simple oils, sometimes with an essential oil added, make decent skin moisturizers.

Don't overdo being clean. Soap and drying of the skin are hard on your skin microorganisms. Use plain soap and don't be obsessive about being clean. Your skin oil is meant to help your skin.

Put a filter on your shower head if you use tap water. Try not to bathe in chlorinated water.

Self-massage with an Ayurvedic sesame oil formula is very beneficial for the skin. Dr. Douillard's website has video instructions for self-massage and sells a nice oil; see the link to his site in the Resources. Feed your skin and support its microbiota.

∾

Microbiota: Gut

Your gut microorganisms perform many vital functions, and how you treat them determines 85% or more of your overall health.

Don't ingest toxins like pesticides, heavy metals and chemical preservatives. Eat organic, unprocessed foods.

Take probiotics if you have a gut imbalance, after taking antibiotics or after any insult to your gut, such as an illness that involves your gut. Periodically, take a good probiotic just on principle.

Better yet, ferment organic foods from the local market, as in most cases, that is far cheaper and more diverse and helpful than taking a supplement. Fermenting isn't that hard to learn. The one lesson I learned the hard way is that local, organic food is best. Many of the organic foods at a grocery store not only lack the local gut microorganisms you need; they have mold, and it is hard to ferment moldy produce. Fermented foods may not set well with you if you have a histamine sensitivity, but if you balance the cause of that condition, eventually you should be able to eat fermented foods.

It is true that just trying to eat foods the gurus say are good for you can be a challenge if your gut is way out of balance, so balance it first, using the suggestions in the previous section of this chapter.

Your vagus nerve, the longest cranial nerve that wanders through your body, has a close relationship with many functions, among them, your digestion. If your vagus nerve is not performing well, you will have signs of digestive problems and also possibly symptoms like inflammation, chronic fatigue and depression. Often, people will go to a doctor with a symptom that is caused by a problem with the vagus nerve and end up with a prescription for erasing that symptom. It is better if you make sure your vagus nerve is able to do its job well.

Support the function of your vagus nerve by lowering stress, doing toning, deep breathing and other natural techniques. If you have vagus nerve symptoms, reducing caffeine, alcohol and stress are helpful. Vagus nerve issues can contribute to health anxiety, as the symptoms are troubling, but anxiety then contributes to trouble with the vagus nerve. Reducing stress and anxiety is helpful to your health in general and for the vagus in particular. Do some online research about the vagus nerve and make sure yours is healthy and balanced.

If you are looking for one place to start building the best health possible, your gut is an excellent place to begin.

~

Detoxification

There are two ways to deal with toxins: avoid them or detoxify after exposure. The best option is to avoid exposure. Toxins tax your system, and dealing with them post-exposure can be difficult. This is especially true for heavy metals like mercury and lead, glyphosate, which is in most foods that aren't organic, and non-native EMFs.

Avoid toxic drinks and food, cosmetics and personal care products and toxic environments like non-native EMFs.

If you are unavoidably exposed to toxins, you can sometimes use activated charcoal or bentonite clay internally to help chelate the toxins. This won't work for everything, but it is a useful periodic strategy. We've also done clay baths for that purpose.

Your liver takes care of detoxification, and the herb milk thistle is often used to help the liver repair. If you have liver issues or a toxic lifestyle, dowse or check with your holistic practitioner about the use of milk thistle. There are other herbs if milk thistle doesn't test well for you.

Oil pulling is an ancient Indian practice that is healing and detoxifying, plus it's simple. Most people use coconut or sesame oil for oil pulling. You can google and see if it resonates with you. It is also very beneficial for the health of teeth and gums and can resolve a number of symptoms.

Proper breathing is very detoxifying. Study and practice a breathing exercise like alternate nostril, circular or deep breathing. Many toxins are removed from your body if you breathe effectively. It has been proven in studies that nostril breathing is far healthier than mouth breathing. Try to breathe through your nose at night and during exercise.

Massage and sauna are two wonderfully natural detoxifying methods that can also be used for maintaining good health. Studies now confirm that sweating detoxifies heavy metals and at least some petrochemicals and pesticides, so sauna therapy is worth exploring.

Fasting has also been shown to be excellent for detoxification, but if you are highly toxic, consult a holistic practitioner first.

Your lymphatic system is vital for the removal of waste products and toxins from your body. A sedentary lifestyle leads to an unhealthy lymphatic system. It's very important to move your body to help the lymph flow and do its job. Walking is excellent for this purpose, as is rebounding, which can be done inside in any weather using a small mini-trampoline. Dr. Axe (link in the Resources section) has a nice article on his website on the benefits of rebounding and how to select a good rebounder. Getting one secondhand can be an inexpensive but valuable investment.

Your thoughts are the most potentially toxic things that affect your health. Learn to monitor your thoughts and focus on what you want, not what you fear or don't want or cannot control. Catch yourself saying toxic things like, "My back is killing me," or "That's going to ruin my health." If you must eat fast food occasionally or travel through a high-EMF zone, do NOT think negative thoughts. Think of how safe and protected you are. This is where intention works best with an anchor of some sort, as in the case of wearing a crystal like shungite or a color or symbol or something else that you feel is protective.

There is no way to avoid all toxins, but you can take action to mitigate the effects and avoid the worst ones if you live more naturally. It is wise to detoxify regularly, and since each method has its own strengths, it is a good idea to employ a variety of detoxification strategies and rotate them or dowse when to use each one, so that you get optimal results.

~

EMFs

It is getting harder and harder to avoid non-native EMFs, but you can take steps to reduce your exposure. In terms of what you can do to mitigate the effects of non-native EMFs, the following are a good starting point:

- Convert your wifi to an ethernet connection
- Avoid smart appliances and meters or deactivate their RF (radio frequency) activity
- Swap your smart phone for a flip phone
- Check your home for dirty electricity or have a professional do it. Then fix it as best you can.
- Make sure your bedroom is free of electrosmog. Remove TVs, phone chargers and clock radios (especially if close to the bed). Make it an EMF-free zone if possible.
- Get rid of your microwave. Use a toaster oven instead
- Never carry or wear devices that put out any non-native EMFs
- Get rid of your tablet, Kindle and other similar devices
- Avoid work situations that bathe you in non-native EMFs
- Use a blue light filtering program or eyeglasses when you must stare at screens
- Limit exposure to blue light to mornings if possible; eliminate it in evenings altogether

- Avoid the use of electric lighting after sunset; use oil lanterns instead
- Use a method of protection that resonates with you, such as wearing a crystal like hematite or shungite with intention

In terms of remediating the effects of exposure to radiation, shungite water has been shown to be useful. Shungite water is made from a unique mineral found only in Russia that has been shown to help with exposure to radiation and EMFs. See the Resources section for the source of shungite we recommend, as not all shungite makes good shungite water. If you have had radiation therapy or exposure to EMFs, the periodic use of shungite water may help with repair. Shungite can also be worn to give some measure of protection against EMFs, though for most, it won't make you bulletproof.

Another promising line of research suggests that some types of mushrooms may heal radiation damage. Chaga has shown promise in offering healing and protection from radiation side effects.

It makes logical sense to have a strong immune system overall in order to react well to environmental challenges, so do your best to foster a healthy immune system.

∽

Body Consciousness

As we have pointed out, your body is an amazing universe composed of trillions of cells, microorganisms and energies. As complex as it is, there are some simple truths about how to best care for it. Most of these suggestions can be implemented by you at little or no cost. Check out the Resources section for some books we like that will help you.

The first step in body consciousness is to actually be in your body and grounded. A huge number of people have adapted to living basically out of body as a survival technique that came in response to trauma or ongoing stress. If you are not in your body, or if you are poorly grounded, you may tend to be spacey, have a high pain threshold, or healing methods don't seem to work on you, or you tend to be more concerned with what others think and want than what you want. You might even find that you don't talk or focus much on yourself at all. If these symptoms describe you, it would be good to dowse if your spirit is out of your body or at least do simple grounding exercises and use intention to bring it back into your body.

Intention is usually enough to bring your spirit back into your body. Just tell it to go back in. But if you are out of body because of ongoing stress, you need to address the cause, or you'll just slip out again. And, be aware that you have this tendency when under stress and instruct your spirit to get back in the body.

It will help if you can do something to reduce fear, like a tapping therapy or the Emotion Code to reduce the stress in your life. Also, it is important to stop thinking of yourself as a powerless victim. Dowsing is the best way to discover if your spirit is out of your body, but if you think it may be the case, using intention to restore it cannot hurt.

A lack of grounding is more common than the spirit being out of the body, but it has some of the same symptoms. Grounding exercises are easy to do and involve visualization. Find one you like on the internet and practice it regularly. If you can dowse, you can determine how well grounded you are on a scale of 0 to 10. It is important to be grounded if you want to have a pleasant and healthy life experience.

How you hold your body also matters. Many of the activities we perform warp our body's natural straight posture, and that is compounded by nutritional and energetic issues and disease symptoms like pain and arthritis. The Alexander Technique is a good starting place for finding out the best way to stand, walk and hold your body. There are many books on the subject, and you can even consult a professional. We like the basis of this method, because it appeals to what is natural for the body.

Moving your body is a natural way to help your health. The lymphatic system needs a certain amount of activity to help move the sludge out of your system. Walking is the best way to get this kind of motion. For most people, it is the least likely to have negative side effects and the easiest to do, because your body was made to walk.

Walking in Nature is even better than mall walking or walking on an indoor track. Your body makes vitamin D from sunlight, and being in Nature has many valuable benefits that have not yet been proven by modern science.

Rebounding is another low impact method that helps your lymphatic system, and it can even be cardiovascular; you can find a used rebounder on Craigslist, and it's something you can do year round inside, regardless of weather.

There are many self-massage techniques that are highly beneficial. Dr. Douillard's website has a great video on an Ayurvedic self-massage technique, as does Agustoni's book listed in the Resources section.

~

Sleep

Sleep is vital to your health. Of the small number of factors that we know affect sleep in a negative way, certain foods, EMFs and stress are the best three places to start for improving your ability to get the healthful rest you need.

Don't eat in the three hours before bedtime.

Avoid caffeine, sugar and alcohol late in the day. Eat a good natural diet that promotes proper melatonin levels.

Don't use electric lights after sunset. Use oil lanterns or something similar.

Do not stare at any kind of screen after sunset or in the two or three hours before bedtime. Use filters or glasses as appropriate the rest of the day. Limit all screen staring, because there are no perfect fixes.

Reduce stress in your life. Take up meditation, guided visualizations or have a hot soak before bedtime. Use lavender essential oil in your bath and drink chamomile tea before bed. Do whatever it takes to set aside worry and stress so you can get a good night's rest.

Most of these suggestions are not costly in terms of money, but they require a commitment to change your behavior. Yet isn't it true that changing your behavior is necessary if you want different outcomes? Just do it.

~

Breathing

How you breathe has a surprisingly large impact on your health, so it is a great place to start your new health regimen, because it costs you absolutely nothing and will immediately yield benefits.

You probably are aware that shallow breathing isn't that healthy, and that breathing not only oxygenates your blood, but releases toxins, performing a vital role for your health. But there is so much more that breathing does for you, if you do it optimally.

Some of the benefits of deep breathing, when done through the nose, are:

- Boosting nitric oxide, which improves the immune system and has many other health benefits, possibly even helping you to lose unwanted weight
- Balancing the vagus nerve, which affects digestion, stress reduction and helps the brain communicate with the gut
- Activating the parasympathetic nervous system, balancing blood pressure and helping with mood stability
- Improving athletic performance
- Improving brain wave coherence
- Boosting alpha wave activity in the brain
- Improving lower lung gas exchange
- Increasing endurance
- Decreasing stress during exercise

Training yourself to nose breathe rather than mouth breathe at night will decrease snoring and possibly even help you reach deep sleep more easily, and some studies suggest you will get sick less often if you nose breathe, probably due to the release of nitric oxide.

There are a number of different breathing techniques that employ deep breathing: alternate nostril breathing and circular breathing may be familiar to you, but have you heard of Brahmari pranayama (pranayama is the name for all deep breathing techniques in Ayurveda)? This technique is deep breathing through the nose combined with humming on the out breath. Brahmari pranayama is easy to do and has been shown to release 15X more nitric oxide than gentle nose breathing. So combining deep breathing with nose breathing and humming is a powerful technique. It's easy to do, and you can visit Dr. John Douillard's website to watch a video on how to do it. See the link in Resources.

Toning is a simple healing and balancing method that uses sound and breathing to stimulate the body's self-healing response. Anyone can learn to tone with very little investment of time or money. Laurel E. Keyes wrote the classic book on this technique, and an updated version has been published with Don Campbell called *Toning: The Healing Power Of The Voice.*

One of the best places to make changes in your health regimen is to improve your breathing. It costs nothing but a little awareness and effort, and yet yields fabulous benefits.

~

Your Subtle Energy Body

Attending to the condition of your subtle energy body is not optional. Trying to create good health only by doing physical things is a waste of time and money, as many people learn the hard way. If you have certain negative beliefs, chakra imbalances or your spirit is out of your body, all the supplements and treatments in the world will not give you the health you want.

Back when we worked with clients, it was not that rare for a client to confess they had invested thousands of dollars trying to find a way to overcome a health challenge, with no lasting results. One client said she had invested $100,000 in her health and was not getting positive outcomes.

Evaluate your health and your health goals. If you have a longstanding problem or you are not getting good results in spite of investing in outside help, therapies and products, it is probably because you have an energy-related condition that you need to address as a root cause.

Energy problems are harder to deal with, because they are basically invisible, and it is hard to find a good practitioner to work with who can honestly tell you whether their approach is going to help you. Any kind of energy therapy is helpful, so it isn't a waste like throwing supplements at something can be, but it is most effective if you can address YOUR core issue specifically.

There is no easy way for us to guide you in this search, but being aware will help you. If you can dowse, that will help you choose an effective path or method. Your intuition speaks for your body's native intelligence, if you can learn to be aware of what it is trying to tell you. So even if you are not a dowser, focusing on developing an awareness of your intuition will help you find a more successful path to your health goals.

The following basic subjects are worth addressing, no matter what your health challenges or condition:

- Chakra balancing
- Grounding
- Setting of good boundaries and reducing empathy
- Keeping your spirit in your body
- Getting rid of fear
- Getting rid of health anxiety
- Learning to be happy
- Getting rid of false subconscious beliefs and programming

There are simple methods you can use, most of which require little financial investment, for doing the above. Some examples include:

- Meditation
- Toning
- Chakra work
- Grounding exercises
- Deep breathing exercises
- Becoming more aware and grateful for what you have
- Tapping therapies like EFT (Emotional Freedom Technique)
- Law of Attraction work
- Energy methods like Tai Chi and Chi Gong

Many of the above can be learned easily via books, online programs or DVDs, all of which are small investments. Working on beliefs and programming is a more complex topic, and like dowsing, will require training or hiring a professional, but they are worth investing in.

The health of your energy body, and your mental/emotional well-being are the foundation of your physical health, so you really need to put effort into them.

∽

Healing & Self-Care

There are too many healing and self-care methods to give them all proper mention in this guide, but we will mention a few that we have used with success over the years. Bear in mind that no healing method cures everything or works for everyone. Your unique frequency will respond best to a method that resonates with it, and as you change and heal, you may find it useful to change methods.

Self-care is the foundation of prevention. By eating well, getting enough sleep, monitoring your thoughts and taking care of yourself, you will need less intervention by professionals. We have found that having a toolbox of several modalities is best. For us, the Emotional Freedom Technique (EFT) has been useful for many situations that relate to emotional trauma and energies. Simple methods like toning, meditation and breathing exercises cost very little and are easy to learn, and we highly recommend them to everyone.

There are many energy healing methods like Reiki, Jin Shin Jyutsu and Spiritual Healing. Most require that you obtain proper training and practice, and none of them cures everything. But it is good to have at least one healing method you can use for self-care.

When healing an existing situation, you may need outside help. A holistic practitioner who uses herbs, homeopathic, chiropractic, cranial sacral therapy and other methods can help you restore balance to your body so you can take over the self-care with little input from professionals.

Healing can take a long time if you are trying to resolve a longstanding issue. You may have to consult different professionals and explore various methods to find what works for you, just as you do with self-care.

Just remember to do everything with intention. Focus on what you are creating, not what you want to eradicate. Take time to gather tools that appeal to you for healing and self-care, and try to enjoy the journey of self-discovery. We have listed some resources in that section of the book.

∽

Your Environment

Your environment has a big effect on your health on all levels. Here are some tips for helping you to create better health by choosing healthier environments:

1. Avoid forms of entertainment that are ugly, scary or engender negative emotions
2. Do regular space clearings on your home and workspace (see the Resources section for a link to our books on space clearing at http://sixthsensebooks.com)
3. Eat good, organic unprocessed foods with positive intentions, gratitude and love
4. Limit your exposure to news, social media and other information outlets which mostly promote fear, overwhelm and negativity
5. Spend time in Nature regularly
6. Avoid people who are toxic
7. Get out of working situations that are toxic

8. Downsize your financial obligations to give yourself more freedom of choice

By simplifying and harmonizing your outer environment, you create the space to build good health.

Your external environment is actually a good snapshot of what your own energies and active beliefs are at any given time. If you are not happy with your external environment or feel it is impacting you detrimentally, it will be useful to address your own beliefs, emotions and behaviors to help shift negative energies in your environment.

∿

Beliefs, Thoughts & Emotions

As you imagine and visualize and verbalize your new story, in time you will believe the new story, and when that happens, the evidence will flow swiftly into your experience. A belief is only a thought you continue to think; and when your beliefs match your desires, then your desires must become your reality.

There is no physical body, no matter what the conditions, that cannot achieve an improved condition. Nothing else in your experience responds as quickly as your own physical body to your patterns of thought.

Excerpted from Money and the Law of Attraction on 8/31/08

Your thoughts are the most important tool for creating the health you want. What you think, what you believe, you experience. You may object to this statement, especially if you consciously do everything you can to create good health, but aren't experiencing it. But let's start here, because not all people consciously are thinking positive thoughts about health.

If you go around calling a disease or pain 'yours', that is counterproductive and identifies it as a part of you. "My back is killing me" or "my diabetes" are not helpful things to think or say. If you find yourself identifying with pain or disease, your thought process is contributing to the problem, not solving it. Recognizing that a negative experience is not an integral part of who you are is an empowering first step towards better health.

What if you already know not to do this, and you are doing your best to make good choices for your health goals, but you still struggle to get results? There are a number of possible issues at work.

Most people who follow the Law of Attraction have problems making it work, because it's all about your vibration, which is the sum total of your conscious and subconscious beliefs, traumas and thoughts. People don't understand that your subconscious has more control over your creative process than your conscious mind. It can be very challenging to reveal road bumps that are subconscious, but they have a huge impact on your health. Dowsing is the best way we know of revealing your subconscious beliefs, but if you observe your life carefully, you can tell what you believe, because what you are experiencing now is in alignment with your vibration.

That can really be a shock, but it's a wakeup call. If you aren't experiencing a healthy, comfortable life now, it's time to change your vibration. The first step in that process is releasing fear. Fear blocks intuition and does you absolutely no good at all. There are many ways to release fear, from tapping (like EFT) to The Emotion Code to simply meditating. Choose one that works for you.

A quick Jin Shin Jyutsu fix for fear is to wrap the fingers of one hand around the index finger of the other and hold it while breathing slowly and deeply in and out, paying attention only to your breathing. Then switch after a while and do the other index finger. This works so well, you can feel the fear draining away. We've put a link in the Resources to a website that gives illustrations and instructions.

Start your day by focusing on what you intend to create and being grateful for your many blessings. End each day by reviewing the good things that have happened and being grateful for them. What you focus on expands, so this is a useful exercise.

～

The Placebo Effect

The Placebo effect is underrated and under-researched in our opinion, as it is the manifestation of your body's natural ability to heal itself with nothing other than positive expectations and focus. How effective has the placebo effect been shown to be in scientific studies? A cursory examination on Google reveals rates as high as 62% for the success of the placebo effect, though the average rates seem to be lower.

If you can persuade someone to be cured without any actual treatment in even 30% of cases, why hasn't anyone done more study on this remarkable phenomenon, which has no side effects? Because there is no way to control or monetize it. Yet those facts make it the perfect therapy for you on your path to health empowerment.

We have a link in the Resources to Dr. Joe Dispenza's book on this subject, and it's a great place to start learning how to harness the power of your mind to allow the body's natural intelligence to kick in and heal and balance.

Dr. John Douillard discusses on his website that he postulates that focusing on taking a pulse, as is done in Ayurvedic and Oriental medicine, can trigger the body's natural healing abilities in some cases, he believes by increasing self-awareness, which is a purpose of Ayurveda. If so, it is probably because of the focus at the time. I have found that doing the jin shin finger holds and the cranial sacral exercises covered in the self-help book we recommend in the Resources both have noticeable and almost immediate positive effects. So it is possible that there are a number of simple things you can do to tap into the placebo effect, but what they have in common is focus, emptying the mind of other things, self-awareness and openness/allowing.

Dowsing is about emptying your mind of everything except your dowsing question and allowing the answer to come to you. In a similar way, focusing on your pulse or awareness of your body while emptying your mind of all else perhaps makes you receptive to the body's ability to restore balance and harmony, perhaps opening you to healing rather than answers, as dowsing does.

The placebo effect is powerful and not well understood, but it is worth researching. Many of the simpler methods we recommend could be used as doorways to increased self-awareness and harnessing the placebo effect.

∿

Exercise

You can't change everything at once. Pick what areas you feel will be easiest to change. That's right. Don't set yourself up for failure by trying to do too much or trying to change things that are too big for you to change at this time. Slow, stepwise change is good. Make it a journey, not a rush to a destination. Allow yourself to take three steps forward and one back. You are still going to make noticeable progress. People too often sabotage themselves by trying to change too much, too fast, then end up right back where they started.

1. What feels like the easiest change to make for you in terms of investment and belief?
2. How strongly do you believe you can make positive changes in that?

3. How will you measure change? (Having more energy, feeling happier and more content, etc)

4. How will you go about making the change? What methods or modalities will you use?

5. Remember that whatever you do, do it with positive intention. Don't make it another task on your already busy calendar. Expect positive results and be patient. Enjoy learning as you go.

8

IT'S YOUR CHOICE

Make Conscious Choices

Envision yourself living naturally. What does that mean to you?
Think about your ideal environment. In this case, 'environment'
includes home, work, relationships with family and friends, your
spiritual beliefs and the energies associated with them and how
comfortable you are in expressing them.

Part of natural health is to nurture yourself with supportive
environments. This means have a job you love, or at the very least,
one that is not horribly stressful. If your job doesn't pay well, has a
lot of responsibility, terrible hours and exposes you to toxic
environments, something is wrong. You cannot expect good health if
you stay in a bad job. Your health is your first priority, so get a new
job as needed, even if it means giving up some material comforts.

Do you live in a toxic neighborhood with gang shootings or lots of
crime? Are you surrounded by non-native EMFs that you cannot
control? Some environmental energies—the ones that are not
ongoing—can be cleared by using space clearing methods. But
ongoing toxic issues cannot easily be dealt with. Moving is your best

solution. It comes to choices, and your health needs to be your top priority.

What if you are in an abusive relationship or your family is very negative towards you, constantly draining your energy and never giving back? How you interact with others affects your health. Toxic relationships that involve being a doormat, letting psychic vampires drain your energy or allowing yourself to be mistreated will have a very bad effect on your health. In many cases, relationship challenges are related to ancestral patterns. They can be challenging to deal with, but it is imperative you do so.

There is always a choice. We all have free will, but often, we don't exercise it for one reason or another. Money, status and approval are not as important as your health. Or, at least, we'd like you to feel that way. You can choose an unhappy but financially wealthy marriage or a career that grinds you down, though it lets you live rather well, but is that what you consciously want? Do you want to suffer in order to have stability or approval or status? Is your health not worth more than that?

We don't claim the choices are always easy. If they were, everyone would choose wisely. But recognizing you do have a choice is the first step in taking measures to improve your life and create the health you want.

～

Dependents: Children & Pets

If you have dependents, your choices and example have a great effect on their health. It can be very challenging to buck a trend, like to refuse vaccinations or fight EMFs in schools. Your kids won't appreciate you saying they should eat good food when their friends are eating junk, because they don't have the information or big picture you do. Your children will be upset if you limit TV or computer time, because once again, they want to do what their friends do. God forbid you don't let them have a smartphone...

It can be stressful to create a safe and healthy environment for your children. You have to pick your battles and do the best you can, always saying out loud that this is for their health and well-being, even if they cannot understand. And you must give good example. Practice what you preach.

Fortunately, pets don't compare notes with other pets. However, you may still be under pressure by friends, the media and veterinarians to do things you don't feel are safe. Chipping your pet, vaccinating frequently, feeding processed food and exposing them to EMFs with radio collars have side effects. Pets have the same health challenges as owners. We are making the same mistakes in their diet, exercise and health care that we make with ourselves. It is up to you to decide what to do.

I recall my mother making some choices about my health when I was young for which I have always been grateful. She was willing to buck health care professionals when she intuitively felt their suggestions were a mistake. For a long period of time when I was young, I was ill a lot, and my blood values were very strange. I remember feeling I had turned into a pincushion, so many samples had been taken, and yet no diagnosis was found. At last, in desperation, the doctors wanted to do a bone marrow test—I think they suspected something like leukemia—and my mother refused to subject me to that. Somehow, she just knew it wasn't the right way to go. And she was correct. Later, when I was a teenager, the orthodontist suggested the best way to straighten my teeth was to surgically remove part of my upper jaw in addition to regular orthodontics. My mother put her foot down on that.

My Mom had no medical training, but was highly intuitive, and she was also very protective. I look back on those times and realize she saved me from unnecessary pain and suffering by saying no to the 'experts.' She is an example to me of how we must all listen to our own intuition, not blindly do whatever we are told.

It all comes down to choice, and when you are in a position of making an unpopular choice, bucking a trend or going against what loved ones want, it can be very challenging. All we can say is do your best to live in accordance with your beliefs. That is integrity. When your children grow up and move out, they can make their own choices, but your dependents rely on your helping them to stay healthy, so make the best choices you can.

∾

Be Empowered

How much and what you do with the information in this book is up to you. You have the right to live your life in the best way you can. But it isn't easy to take an unconventional path. Peer pressure is as powerful and as negative as your mother warned you, and it continues long after you leave school.

The media, friends and family and some of the people in positions of power will apply pressure to you if you want to think outside the box and live more naturally. You may find yourself the subject of derision or even verbal attacks.

The thing to remember is that although you are acting in an unconventional way, you are not alone. There is plenty of support out there, and it is wise to mingle with those who see things your way. In this section, we address some of the more common negative behaviors you may encounter on your journey, with ideas for how to deal with them in a positive fashion and still feel comfortable with your choice.

∾

You're Not Stupid

Plenty of people are into DIY (do-it-yourself), because it saves money and because they like to do things themselves. You don't see across-the-board scoffing at DIY. Home Depot and Lowe's make a ton of money off people doing DIY projects.

Successful DIYers aren't derided, yet most people who would not hesitate to try and replace a doorknob or wire an outlet are horrified at the prospect of caring for their own health. Why is that? Getting a medical degree is expensive, time-consuming and takes a certain level of intelligence, so doctors get an automatic level of respect that reflects their investment. Yet they are not really that different from a competent and masterful plumber, electrician or auto mechanic. Specialized knowledge is valuable, and it seems that modern life has proliferated lots of specialties that didn't exist up until recent time.

One hundred or more years ago, families usually cared for their own health except in extreme conditions. There were many home remedies that used natural things like plants to treat symptoms and conditions. As life became more complicated and introduced other factors to challenge health—remember the term 'diseases of civilization'— people looked for magic bullets. Penicillin and cortisone are examples of discoveries that were hailed as miracles. While they provided benefits, it turned out there were side effects. As we pointed out, humans aren't very good about caution or admitting how little they know.

Any given doctor or researcher only knows a small percent of the entire body of biological knowledge, so don't let anyone make you feel stupid just because you didn't go to med school or don't have a degree in science. I have two degrees in Biology, and I can tell you that what I have learned in my post-college years by studying on my own has given me far more useful knowledge than I got in college. College to me was more of an opportunity to learn how to research and where to look for knowledge and how to think critically. You can't teach everything about a topic in four to six years. You just can't. Yet after college, it has been shown that very few people even read on a regular basis. It's as if leaving school means they know it all. This is an unfortunate but common misconception.

Most doctors are so overworked that they have little free time to keep up with recent developments (in 2015 alone, 806,000 papers were indexed at the National Library of Medicine), so they just parrot what they learned in school, or in some cases, as with nutrition, what they didn't learn.

Another factor is on your side. Your body knows what it needs, and you have an intimate familiarity with it that gives you a perspective no doctor could ever have. Don't discount that. Combined with your intuition, that gives you an advantage no health care provider has.

You have a great deal to contribute to your healing process. You can learn how to care for yourself, and when you need outside assistance, you can participate in the process. Don't give your power away.

Critical thinking, like intuition, is a tool you can use that will help you reach your health goals. Critical thinking doesn't mean being negative. It means you find out the facts for yourself before making a decision.

One of the goals of this book is to give you a background in how to think logically about health and how to ask questions and make decisions that make sense, rather than just following the crowd or doing what you are told. This is the value of critical thinking. It is a tool for making good decisions using your rational mind, just as dowsing is a tool for making good choices using your intuition.

~

Critical Thinking Examples

Instead of simply doing what the media or your doctor or friend says, we feel you will get better results if you think before taking action that affects your health.

Here are some questions to ask about situations, products, procedures and lifestyle choices:

- Is it natural? Be sure you define natural well.
- If not, has it really been proven to be safe? Just because someone says it is safe does not mean anything.
- If not, who benefits from not testing it? Why would they take a chance on finding out it's dangerous? Why pay to find that out? Who else has the money to test it? What happens if no one is interested in funding tests?
- Are there any laws indemnifying the makers/sellers? This is generally a bad sign. Good products and procedures thrive in capitalist societies. The bad ones are supposed to flop, not be protected from lawsuits and failure.
- How are those who disagree painted in the media? Are there professionals and people of stature who are being attacked, slandered or losing their jobs because they object to a certain product or practice? Are people considered freaks and conspiracy theorists to be against it? Ad hominem tactics (attacking the person, not their arguments) like that are used when someone has a weak position or the truth is not on their side.
- Who benefits most from selling this product? Are they against testing? Do they paint objections as stupid? Making fun of a position is not necessary if you are in the right.

These are questions to ask yourself in order to make a good decision. Make choices based on what you believe will serve your health in the long run. There will always be new things to decide about; get an approach that works for you.

~

It's Just A Choice

Ultimately, all of life is a choice. You have free will and the right to exercise it. You can choose whatever lifestyle suits you. Don't regard things as either black and white. Don't judge your choices. Just do what you think is best, keep learning—because there is so much left to discover—and adjust as you learn more.

Don't be upset with yourself if you can't make all the choices you want, because of money or some other obstacle. Don't feel victimized by other people's choices.

Do not allow others to try and convince you that you should not exercise your free will.

Health, like life, is a journey, and you have a right to choose what you think is best for your health goals. Focus on what you can do, improve things as you go and grant others the right to choose for themselves.

~

Responding To Skeptics

Not everyone has the same beliefs. When you face skeptics, be aware that they aren't looking for the truth. They aren't looking to change. It can be very unpleasant talking with someone who believes the opposite of what you believe. Yet sometimes, you may feel the need to interact with a skeptic.

When someone attacks you or puts you down for your beliefs, they will usually say one of a few things:

- There's no proof/studies showing what you say is true/that it is dangerous
- That's just silly nonsense
- We've been using/doing _____for years, and no one has shown it is dangerous
- That's not supported by science
- Some will even be angry, which is another sign that they don't have a leg to stand on and don't want you to exercise free will

Give the person a chance to show whether they are just parroting something they've heard or they really have researched. In almost all cases, they will merely be repeating what they've heard. Don't accuse them; ask them meaningful questions that allow them to expound on their beliefs. If they have really thought about the subject, they will have interesting answers, but most won't be able to answer questions like these:

"Oh, have you done a lot of searching on Google for studies and found none?"

"Where did you hear that?"

"What makes you say that?"

"How is it not scientific?"

"Could you explain what you mean by that?"

"What books or studies have you read that support that?"

"Can I send you some links to studies/etc?"

Ask questions and be open to hearing answers, but don't expect any that make sense, because most people are not speaking from knowledge; they are speaking from fear, ignorance and prejudice. No one wants to feel like an outcast, so objectors are made to feel like freaks. But most people in favor of these things are just repeating what the media says. They have not spent even one minute thinking.

If they are open, offer to email them some links to research, book titles or websites that have useful information. Show that you aren't combative, that you're happy to share what you've learned. See the Resources for examples. More resources are coming along all the time.

Whatever you do, be patient, ask questions and try to get people to think, to explain in logical terms why they believe what they do. Many will become agitated and angry when pushed that way. Just stay patient and ask questions. They may break off the conversation in anger, but perhaps down the line, they will begin to think about what you have said.

It is impossible to persuade people to your way of thinking. Don't make that your mission. Just be glad you have an open mind and a willingness to learn.

~

Exercise

If you had unlimited time, money and freedom, and you didn't have to answer to anyone, what would you believe and do about your health?

If there is a vast gulf between what you are now doing and what you would prefer to do, do not become discouraged. By identifying how much resistance you have, how blocked you are and where you are blocked or resisting, you pave the way to making positive changes and empowering yourself to experience the health you desire.

9

USING DOWSING & INTUITION

Sometimes you walk into things, that, if you were paying attention, vibrationally, you would know right from the beginning that it wasn't what you are wanting. In most cases, your initial knee-jerk response was a pretty good indicator of how it was going to turn out later. The things that give most of you the most grief are those things that initially you had a feeling response about, but then you talked yourself out of it for one reason or another.

-Abraham Hicks

Intuition is a natural human sensing ability, but most people don't use it to advantage. That's partly because we live in a rational, scientistic society, and intuition is nonlinear and hard to explain. Most conventional people scoff at intuition the way they do about New Age stuff. That's because they are ignorant.

Your intuition gives you an array of information-gathering abilities that you can fine tune to add to the information your physical senses give you, and to back up the analysis of your rational mind. Intuition and rational thinking are complementary. Our culture, unlike native ones, has largely dismissed intuition in favor of rationality, as if you must make a choice.

Living a natural, healthy life is best done by using all of your talents and gifts. Your intuition is a powerful tool for reaching conclusions your brain cannot reach and for guiding you to the best choice when you lack enough rational data.

Your body has a natural intelligence which we have mentioned, and intuition is part of that intelligence. By focusing your intuition, you can get better results than if you neglect your intuition. But how do you do that?

The simplest advice we can give is that you choose to become aware of what your intuition is trying to tell you. You have intuitive senses, and they are always there, at work. But your brain filters the vast amount of information given to you by all your senses, and if you want to tap into your intuition, first you will need to choose to pay attention to it.

This is harder than it sounds, but the good news is anyone can do it. Visit Sixth Sense Books at http://sixthsensebooks.com to see our books on dowsing and intuition.

For us, dowsing was the gateway to a happier, healthier, intuitive lifestyle. Dowsing is a technique for using your intuition combined with your rational mind to get answers to questions your brain cannot answer.

Dowsing is a skill anyone can learn, but like any skill, it takes time and practice to learn proper technique. Complicating that is the fact that each dowsing application is a specialty with its own pitfalls and techniques. It is rare for a dowser to master more than a few dowsing applications.

Health dowsing is a powerful dowsing application and one of the most popular for dowsers. As a dowser, you can:

- Select the best therapy for your health goals
- Measure the side effects of a drug, surgery or technique

- Discover the root cause of a health issue and the best method for remedying it
- Determine how long to apply a particular remedy
- Select a good doctor or healer
- Determine what you are allergic to
- Find out the level of function of your organs, systems, chakras and your aura
- Know when you will most benefit from a detox and what type to use
- And so much more…

Dowsing for health is an application we mastered over many years of working with clients and dowsing for ourselves and our pets, and we love teaching people how to master dowsing and use it to improve their lives. If you are interested in health dowsing, get our book *Dowsing For Health,* as it is a comprehensive training in this valuable topic. However, dowsing isn't for everyone. If you have a quick, rational mind, are verbally gifted and think like an engineer or scientist, dowsing may be perfect for you. If that doesn't sound like you, then another gateway to intuition may appeal more.

Intuition is a knowing that you can tap into so that you make choices that help you reach your goals. Using your intuition is empowering, and it will save you time, effort and money. Check the Resources section for information on our free dowsing website, our books on dowsing and intuition and our dowsing course, because living without using your intuition is laboring under a handicap.

10

SUMMARY

It's easy to suggest that you choose a lifestyle that is in alignment with what Nature designed you for so that you can experience optimal health, but following through is very challenging. We don't realize how many technological advances and conveniences we have accepted as normal that are anything but 'natural.' Yet, if you give up everything that is not natural, how can you expect to live in modern society? You can't.

We aren't suggesting you give up everything. There have been advances in the past hundred years that are wonderful. Not all technological breakthroughs are harmful. But added together, the burden of modern life with its non-native EMFs, toxic drugs, pesticides, stress, negativity and food empty of nutrients adds up to dis-ease, especially as you grow older. It is not a coincidence that degenerative diseases are growing rapidly in spite of everything medical science does.

Ultimately, it's up to each individual to choose their lifestyle. If you choose with eyes open, you can have better health than someone who blindly accepts what is 'normal.' It is not normal to decline with age. You can choose to be healthy throughout your life, enjoying life and making a contribution however you choose.

Don't let fear hold you back. Don't let habit determine the outcome of your health. Make conscious choices. Do a little at a time. Slow is good. Watch for unexpected blessings along the way. Know that each positive choice you make is contributing to good health for you and your family and pets. Don't lament that you can't control or change everything at once. Be patient and try to enjoy the journey.

Creating optimal health and longevity is a big project that will require investment of time and effort on your part, but it will pay you back many times over. You can live a healthier life, and you can even learn to enjoy the process of creating good health.

There is no single prescribed path. You are unique. By applying the suggestions in this book and learning to think for yourself and choosing what makes sense to you, you will avoid many of the pitfalls of modern life in terms of health and well-being.

A valuable tool on your journey is to associate with like-minded people, while accepting there are many right paths. Find those who believe in making conscious and natural health choices.

Question everything, but respect the right of others to choose their own path. Finally, become more self-aware and learn to listen to your intuition, whether you focus by dowsing or access it in another way. Your body has a natural intelligence, the ability to heal itself when given the right conditions.

11

RESOURCES

Thanks to the internet, you have You Tube, books, free webinars and newsletters to pour information directly into your home. When we were young, you had to go to a library to research topics.

The downside of the wealth of information is that not all of it is useful or even true. In this section, we are listing only sources that we have used for ourselves and feel have value. Over time, some of these may disappear.

More Resources are becoming available on a daily basis. Use your intuition and judgment about what to believe and apply. We include our impressions about most of these resources, to help you decide if you want to pursue them. They are organized by topic.

∾

Books By Maggie & Nigel Percy

Visit Amazon to see our books on dowsing, intuition, energy clearing and related topics.

∾

GENERAL NATURAL HEALTH **Resources**

- In 2025, I discovered Dr. Brian Grimm, MD on Substack. His field biology became the foundation for building good health which I believe anyone can benefit from. His ideas are cutting edge and synthesize a revolutionary, natural approach that combines a number of relatively simple actions that can have profound effect on health. I have applied his suggestions and highly recommend them. Although he has plenty to offer free subscribers, it is well worth the small monthly subscription fee to access more in depth help from him.

- Dr. Joseph Mercola has an extensive website at http://mercola.com. His website is a wealth of information, and I have used and benefited from his products. At the time of this writing, he is working on a major book about health problems associated with EMFs which will probably be very well researched; I look forward to reading it. He is always looking for new ways to improve health, and so sometimes he changes his positions on certain subjects (he has admitted this in public presentations). To me, this is a sign of integrity, but as with all sources, you need to test what he offers against your intuition meter. I consider his site one of the best on the internet by a health care professional.

- Dr. Josh Axe has a great website, and it is probably even more easy to digest than Dr. Mercola's. His site is http://draxe.com. Dr. Axe presents material in a very popular science format that anyone can digest quickly. If you have limited time and not so much biology background, he is a great starting point.

- Green Med Info at http://greenmedinfo.com is a huge site run by Sayer Ji, a respected health expert. He has gathered together articles and scientific studies on topics of interest in such a way that it saves you digging through all that's out there. If it's on his site, it's pretty much guaranteed to be accurate. I subscribe to the newsletter, as he has great articles and notification of free events of interest. I also have a paid subscription to this site, and I have found it to be helpful. If you are a practitioner of any kind or are looking for confirmation in the scientific studies, this is the place to go.

- Dr. John Douillard's website is a beautiful balance of free information and intriguing, unique products that focus on Ayurveda and how you can improve your health using the ancient wisdom of this Indian health system. He is especially good at keeping up with recent scientific studies and showing how they support an Ayurvedic perspective. At http://lifespa.com, this site features videos and articles that are very interesting and revealing. Ayurveda gives you a framework for how you think about natural health, and this site is a wealth of useful information. He also has unique products that have good energy.

- The Human Longevity Project is a documentary series with many experts who share breaking knowledge about what factors contribute to good health and longevity. It's a great, informative series. We liked it so much, we bought it. See it here: https://humanlongevityfilm.com/. This video series was informative and inspiring.

- Biochemical pathways posters: http://bit.ly/biochemicalcharts. This site will give you an idea how complex biology is and how little we know.

- Dr. David Brownstein has authored many books on natural health. The two I've read are on iodine and salt, but he has quite a few. His website is http://drbrownstein.com.

∾

THE NEW BIOLOGY

This is a great article to help orient you to the new way of looking at human biology, which is very much in alignment with ancient health wisdom and a natural approach to health:

http://bit.ly/gminewbiology

≈

Diet & Nutrition Books

You're Not Sick, You're Thirsty: Water For Health, For Healing, For Life by F. Batmanghelidj, MD. This is the updated version of his book from the late 90s, and it is an easier read for sure. It will educate you about the critical functions water performs and may even get you to start drinking more water.

Eat Dirt by Dr. Josh Axe. An easy read to help you understand the importance of the gut microbiome and how to strengthen it.

Eat Wheat by Dr. John Douillard is an interesting book that suggests that the problems people have with digesting wheat involve gut microbiome insufficiencies and modern wheat strains in most cases. While those diagnosed with celiac sprue may never be able to eat wheat, many people who are avoiding wheat at this time could heal their gut, rebuild their microbiome and enjoy Einkorn flour products or other ancient grains in moderation.

The Paleo Solution: The Original Human Diet by Robb Wolf is well-written and provides compelling arguments for adopting an ancestral human diet. While you will find most paleo aficionados eat too much meat, the theory behind paleo is sound, if applied in a more natural way, meaning eating the types of foods in the amounts and during the seasons humans evolved to eat them.

Epi-Paleo Rx by Dr. Jack Kruse is a bit hard to read, but it makes some very good arguments for both ancestral diets and for reducing or eliminating exposure to blue light and electric lights.

Vitamin K2 and the Calcium Paradox by Kate Rheaume-Bleue is a priceless book that should convince you to start supplementing with a good fermented cod liver oil/concentrated butter oil supplement. We simply are not able to eat the foods we did long ago, and we are not getting fat soluble vitamins that are vital for good health.

∾

BOOKS ON SELF-CARE

Body, Breath & Being by Carolyn Nicholls is an excellent self-help book on the Alexander technique, which will help you improve your health and even get rid of symptoms by coordinating various basic body functions in a natural way.

Harmonizing Your Craniosacral System by Daniel Agustoni is a gold mine of simple techniques you can do that will improve your health.

∾

BOOKS On The Subtle Energy Body

Hands Of Light by Barbara Ann Brennan is a good resource for information on evaluating and healing your aura and chakras, as well as including some dowsing techniques for evaluating chakras.

The Subtle Body: An Encyclopedia of Your Energetic Anatomy by Cyndi Dale is comprehensive and very interesting. If you want to learn about the subtle energy body and can only buy one book, this is the one to get.

Karla McLaren's *Your Aura & Your Chakras* is a very useful book for both applying techniques to heal and protect your subtle energy body, but she explains the psychology and personality theory behind various issues, allowing you to see yourself and make some changes to improve the health and balance of your energy body.

The Book of Chakra Healing by Liz Simpson is a nice, comprehensive guide on the chakras and methods for harmonizing them.

∼

SUPPLEMENTS & **Foods**

We supplement all the time with this brand of concentrated butter oil/fermented cod liver oil, because of the fat vitamin deficiencies of a modern diet. It is the brand Green Pasture. http://bit.ly/codbutteroil

We buy kelp products from Maine Coast Sea Vegetables: http://seaveg.com. They can usually be found in whole food stores. We use the seasonings almost daily.

Good salt sources are Celtic Sea Salt and Redmond salt sellers. Himalayan salt is beautiful, but take care of your source, because Chinese products sometimes have heavy metal contamination. We find it useful to alternate products, as they have different trace minerals profiles.

Check out heirloom and ancient grains at these websites:

https://www.einkorn.com/ We've used einkorn flour in moderation and seen my grain symptoms go away.

http://ansonmills.com

http://bit.ly/breadgrains

∼

CANCER

Of great interest to those who take a holistic view is Dr. Hamer's theory on emotional causes of cancer. His theory argues for the necessity of dealing with emotional traumas, because he is totally convinced they lead to cancer if ignored. We urge you to learn EFT or another therapy for clearing emotions and dealing with emotional trauma. Along with your diet, it is a vital factor in your health. His theory can be examined on a number of sites. This is one: http://bit.ly/hamertheory

∽

EMFs

Learn about natural EMF healing and protection via shungite: http://bit.ly/shungitepdf. Also, at http://shungitequeen.com, you can get shungite in various forms, from jewelry to raw elite shungite for making shungite water. Remember protection does NOT mean you should keep being exposed to EMFs, but it can help when you are unable to avoid them.

Dr. Dietrich Klinghardt is a respected authority on EMFs and uses muscle testing as part of his protocols. He has been a guest on a number of documentary series, included some listed here. His website is: https://klinghardtinstitute.com/.

Lloyd Burrell discovered that EMFs were the cause of his health problems, which he subsequently resolved, and he has dedicated himself to educating people about this topic. His website has some good information: https://www.electricsense.com/.

Dr. Martin Pall has contributed to many videos on EMFs that can be seen on You Tube. His work is highly respected.

∽

VACCINATIONS

The best source we have found online is this video series: The Truth About Vaccines. It is well-researched and compelling, and periodically is offered free on various channels. The site is http://thetruthaboutvaccines.com. If you are trying to make your mind up about vaccinations, this is hands down the best current resource available.

A very interesting historical perspective on vaccinations, especially smallpox vaccination in the 19th Century, may be gotten from an extensive publication by Alfred Russel Wallace, co-discoverer with Charles Darwin of the theory of natural selection. Wallace was a highly respected scientist of his times, and reading his work shows that vaccination has never been blindly accepted. If you read his study, you may also then want to google Edward Jenner and learn how he developed the smallpox vaccine. It is nothing short of horrific to modern sensibilities from an ethical and scientific standpoint, yet Edward Jenner is held up as a great scientist of his time. As of this writing, you can access the complete document written by Alfred Russel Wallace online at: http://bit.ly/ wallaceonvax.

∾

THERAPIES

We have studied and been certified in many therapies. What will work best for you depends on your energy, but we love jin shin jyutsu, Emotional Freedom Technique (tapping), meditation and visualization and toning.

Toning and meditation are easy and cheap to learn and practice. EFT has many free resources online and is easy to learn, but you need to be confident verbally to get the most out of it. Jin shin has some very basic techniques you can learn online, and if you like it, invest in a class. It is much more complex, but is based on Oriental medicine.

We have also learned and practiced Reiki, Spiritual Healing, Spiritual Response Therapy and The Emotion Code, but we found ourselves moving on from them after a while.

Jin Shin Jyutsu finger hold instructions and diagrams may be found here: http://bit.ly/jinshinfingers

Breathing exercises are easy to learn and a huge help for building better health. From increasing oxygenation and removing toxins to healing vagus nerve issues, breathing is a free, effective and natural healing and self-care method. You can research online about different techniques or visit Dr. Douillard's website at http://lifespa.com. Just enter terms in the Search box. He has tons of articles and videos.

You might also look into crystal, color and herbal therapies, because they are also natural and effective.

~

PLACEBO EFFECT

Dr. Joe Dispenza's book *You Are The Placebo: Making Your Mind Matter* is a wonderful starting point in learning how to tap into the body's healing intelligence.

~

WATER & Energy

The Hidden Messages In Water by Masaru Emoto is a bestselling book by a Japanese scientist that shows the structure of water changes depending on the type of thoughts directed at it by humans. The micrographs in this book are stunning proof of the ability of water to carry energies. Interestingly, this is one of the reasons that underground water can be noxious. It is also why we avoid using bottled water, as it can pick up energies sitting in a store. However, this research also suggests that you can *change* the energies and structure of water by directing positive thoughts towards it. This gives some support to the idea that saying a blessing over a meal or eating with intention can make your food healing.

The Fourth Phase Of Water: Beyond Solid, Liquid and Vapor by Gerald Pollock presents interesting ideas why we should not regard water as simply a liquid that other stuff in our body is dissolved in. The unique properties of water in biological systems are responsible for health, and there are many factors that affect it, from dehydration to EMF exposure.

∿

Learning To Manifest/Changing Your Outlook

The Law of Attraction is a popular system for manifesting, but it is much more. It is about how your energy and your outlook create your reality. Although we are not big fans of channeled information, the Abraham teachings resonate with us. The main challenge you will have is that even after reading all the books and applying what the website teaches, you may still feel a bit lost as to how to take action to achieve your goals. In spite of that, I have found the material very helpful for reframing what I focus on and taking responsibility for my life experience. You can subscribe and get a free daily quote via email at http://abraham-hicks.com. It's a great starting point, not an end in itself, for creating the life you want.

∿

Fiction Worth Reading

State of Fear by the late Michael Crichton is a great read that relates to how the media is handling vaccination, GMOs and other health issues, though it is on other topics that were current at the time it was written. The principles he expounds in the *Jurassic Park* series and *Next* stimulate a lot of thought about where we are headed as we gain more and more technological and scientific knowledge than we seem capable of handling. In fact, just about anything by Crichton is scientifically solid but honest and cautious about the brave new world science and corporations are trying to create.

PLEASE LEAVE A REVIEW

Our goal was to give you way more value than the price of the book and include all the basics you need to know about natural health, so that you can begin to improve your life.

Please leave a review wherever you purchased this book, because that will help other readers decide if it's for them. Thanks!

OTHER BUSY PERSON'S GUIDES

The Busy Person's Guide To Energy Clearing

The Busy Person's Guide To Space Clearing

The Busy Person's Guide To Ghosts, Curses & Aliens

The Busy Person's Guide: The Complete Series on Energy Clearing

ABOUT MAGGIE & NIGEL PERCY

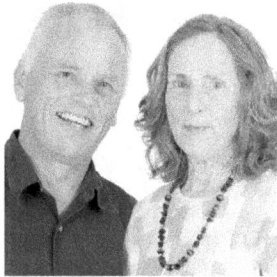

Maggie & Nigel Percy have written over 20 books on dowsing and related topics. Since 2000, they have been teaching and presenting about dowsing, healing, space clearing and other related subjects. For over 15 years, they served a global clientele with dowsing and space clearing services through their business Sixth Sense Solutions. They are now retired and enjoy pursuing their interests to enhance their lives.

www.ingramcontent.com/pod-product-compliance
Lightning Source LLC
Chambersburg PA
CBHW072145270326
41931CB00010B/1894